中等职业教育数字化课程建设教材
供护理、助产及其他医学相关类专业使用

医护英语

YIHU YINGYU

主　编　曹　岚
副主编　梁晓静　宋起慧
编　者（按姓氏汉语拼音排序）
曹　岚（九江市卫生学校）
方　莉（南宁市卫生学校）
黄秋雨（湛江市中医学校）
梁晓静（南宁市卫生学校）
马彦菲（首都医科大学附属卫生学校）
宋起慧（包头市卫生学校）
孙　蔚（九江职业大学）
萧永豪（梧州市卫生学校）
虞文娟（四川护理职业学院）

科学出版社
北　京

内 容 简 介

《医护英语》是为初涉医护专业的中职学生提供的一本学习职场英语的初级教材，是为科学、合理平衡英语和医护专业的教学，满足教师课堂教学而设计的。本教材依托护理基本岗位和职责，以简单的职场英语话题为主线，以任务为导向，辅以功能和结构项目，按照"任务—话题—功能—结构—任务"的格式编排，力求通过反复训练，强化功能表达。同时，学生可学习简单的医护应用文，掌握实用英语写作技巧。本教材旨在对医护专业学生进行听、说、读、写的基础训练，提高医护生对职场英语的运用和理解能力。本教材英语单词约 1 900 个，专业词汇约 200 个；共计 10 个教学单元，每个单元由 Section A，Section B，Section C 三个主要部分构成。总学时为 72，每个单元 5 ~ 7 学时。

本教材可供护理、助产及其他医学相关类专业使用。

图书在版编目（CIP）数据

医护英语 / 曹岚主编. —北京：科学出版社，2018.7
中等职业教育数字化课程建设教材
ISBN 978-7-03-055598-4

Ⅰ. 医… Ⅱ. 曹… Ⅲ. 医学 - 英语 - 中等专业学校 - 教材 Ⅳ. R

中国版本图书馆 CIP 数据核字（2017）第288542号

责任编辑：张立丽 / 责任校对：张凤琴
责任印制：李 彤 / 封面设计：铭轩堂

科学出版社 出版
北京东黄城根北街 16 号
邮政编码：100717
http://www.sciencep.com
北京虎彩文化传播有限公司 印刷
科学出版社发行 各地新华书店经销
*
2018年7月第 一 版 开本：787×1092 1/16
2022年1月第六次印刷 印张：10
字数：238 000
定价：29.80元
（如有印装质量问题，我社负责调换）

中等职业教育数字化课程建设教材

编审委员会

中等职业教育数字化课程建设教材

教材目录

书名	主编	书号
1. 语文	孙敬华　李经春	978-7-03-055597-7
2. 英语	方　莉	978-7-03-055594-6
3. 医护英语	曹　岚	978-7-03-055598-4
4. 计算机应用基础	张全丽	978-7-03-055596-0
5. 职业生涯规划与就业指导	宋晨升	978-7-03-055723-0
6. 护理礼仪	李　蕾	978-7-03-055595-3
7. 人际沟通	王艳华	978-7-03-055397-3
8. 解剖学基础	万爱军	978-7-03-055390-4
9. 生物化学	钟楠楠　丁金娥	978-7-03-055482-6
10. 化学（第3版）	丁宏伟	978-7-03-055914-2
11. 医用物理（第2版）	李长驰	978-7-03-055913-5
12. 生理学基础	柳海滨	978-7-03-055393-5
13. 病理学基础	周士珍　卢桂霞	978-7-03-055395-9
14. 药物学基础	符秀华　付红焱	978-7-03-055387-4
15. 医学遗传学基础	王　懿	978-7-03-055349-2
16. 病原生物与免疫学基础	郑小波　王有刚	978-7-03-055449-9
17. 护理学基础	郭　蔚	978-7-03-055480-2
18. 内科护理	张晓萍	978-7-03-055354-6
19. 外科护理	王　萌　郝　强	978-7-03-055388-1
20. 妇产科护理	李民华	978-7-03-055355-3
21. 儿科护理	李砚池	978-7-03-055394-2
22. 健康评估	袁亚红　程　颖	978-7-03-055391-1
23. 社区护理	马　英	978-7-03-055389-8
24. 老年护理	杨建芬　张　玲	978-7-03-055350-8
25. 传染病护理	曾志励	978-7-03-055720-9
26. 中医护理基础	韩新荣	978-7-03-055558-8
27. 急救护理技术	程忠义	978-7-03-055396-6

前 言 QIAN YAN

党的十九大对优先发展教育事业，加快教育现代化，办好人民满意的教育作出了重要部署，对发展职业教育提出了新的要求——完善职业教育和培训体系，加快实现职业教育的现代化，深化体制机制改革，加强师德建设，深化产教融合、校企合作，提升职业教育开放水平和影响力。为我国新时代职业教育和继续教育指明了方向，明确了任务。

科学出版社深入贯彻党的十九大精神，积极落实教育部最新《中等职业学校专业教学标准（试行）》要求，并结合我国医药职业院校当前的教学需求，组织全国多家医药职业院校编写了全国中等职业教育数字化课程建设规划教材。本套教材具有以下特点：

1. 新形态教材　本套教材是以纸质教材为核心，通过互联网尤其是移动互联网，将各类教学资源与纸质教材相融合的一种教材建设的新形态。读者可通过中科云教育平台，快速实现图片、音频、视频、3D模型、课件等多种形式教学资源的共享，并可在线浏览重点、考点及对应习题，促进教学活动的高效开展。

2. 对接岗位需求　本套教材中依据科目的需要，增设了大量的案例和实训、实验及护理操作视频，以期让学生尽早了解护理工作内容，培养学生学习兴趣和岗位适应能力。教材中知识链接的设置，旨在扩大学生知识面，鼓励学生探索钻研专业知识，不断进步，更好地对接岗位需求。

3. 切合护考大纲　本套教材紧扣最新《护士执业资格考试大纲（试行）》的相关标准，清晰标注考点，并针对每个考点配以试题及相应解析，便于学生巩固所学知识，及早与护考接轨，适应护理职业岗位需求。

《医护英语》是本套教材中的一本，按照本套教材统一要求编写。本教材由10个单元构成。每单元话题设计紧扣医护工作流程，取材实用性强，包括基础护理流程中的接待病人、询问症状及病史、指导就诊、医学检查、打针、用药、办理出入院手续、健教宣传、康复指导等医护场景对话，还包括一些介绍医护科普知识、生活保健常识以及护理史等内容的小文章，突出了医护英语的实用性、科普性、社会性和人文性。本教材配有课文注释、听力原文、课文翻译、单元词汇表、词汇索引表，涵盖了各单元的重点词汇、词组、句型、语法重难点；考虑到当前医护生的英语程度，涵盖了8项基本实用的语法知识。语法内容可供教师根据学生实际情况选择性讲解，也可供医护生根据自己的需要与能力进行学习。此外，教学基本要求、练习题参考答案可供教学参考。

在编写本教程的过程中，编者严谨求实，参阅了大量书籍、网站，并融入了自身教学心得。但由于时间有限，书中的谬误疏漏之处在所难免，敬请读者及同仁批评指正。

编　者

2018年1月

Contents

Unit 1

Welcome to the Nursing School

Section A *My roommate Sarah is in Nursing Class 1.*

Language Goals: Talk about Persons, Places and Studies of Nursing School.

WARM-UP

Ⅰ. Match the phrases with pictures.

________ nurse uniform

________ specimen

________ training classroom

________ nursing trolley

________ nursing school

________ nursing students

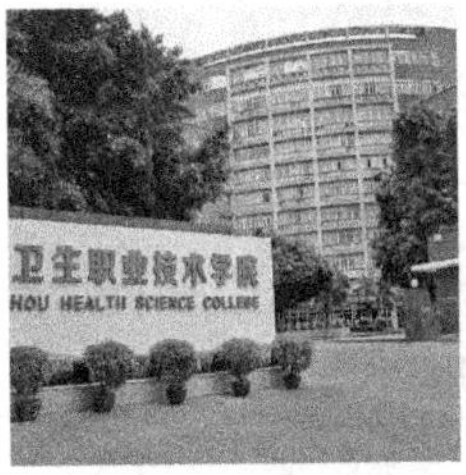

A

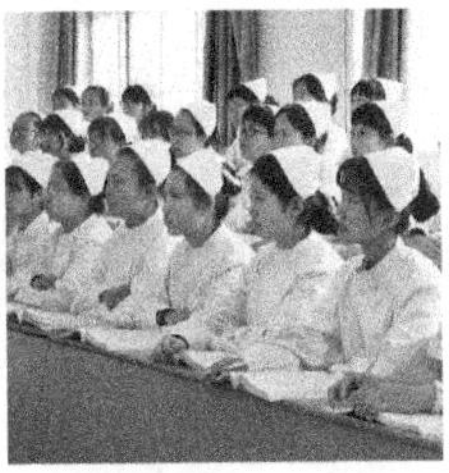

B

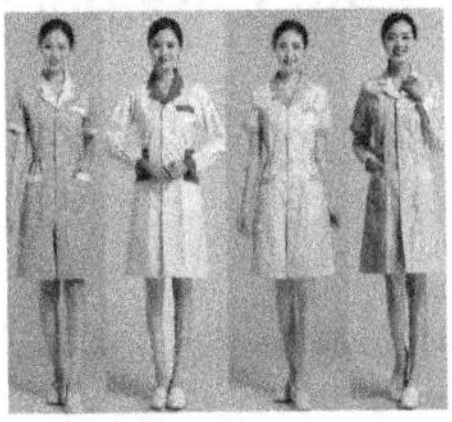

C

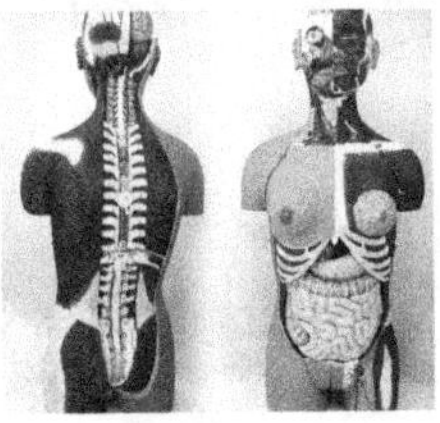

D

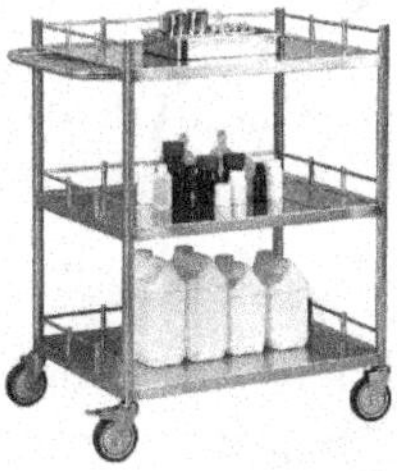

E

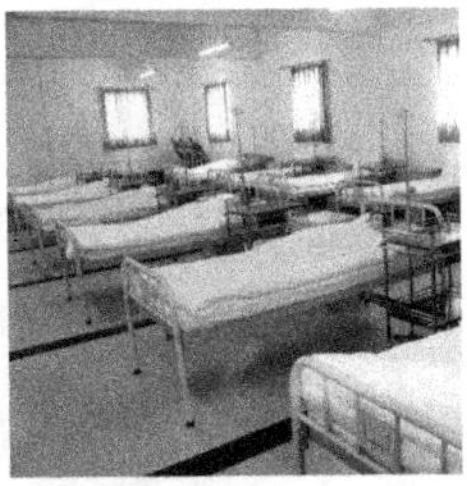

F

Ⅱ. Listen and number the pictures 1 to 4 in the order you hear them.

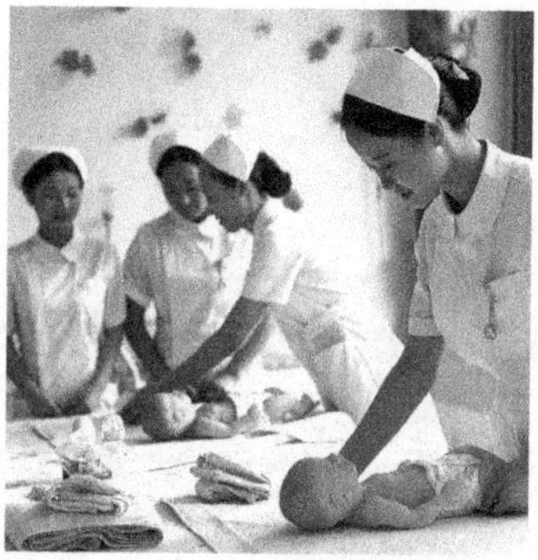

______ have nursing practice class

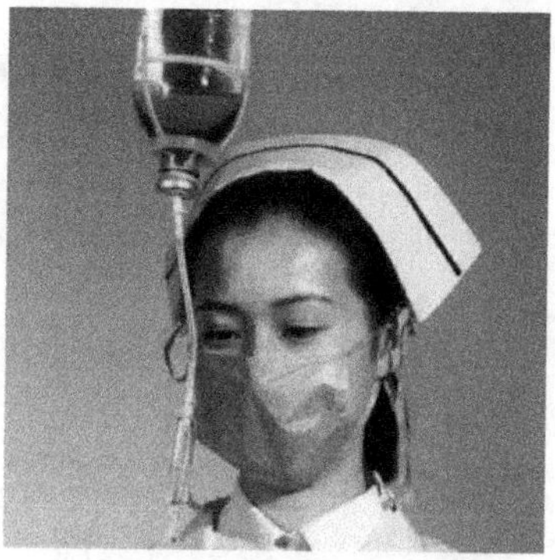

______ give an injection

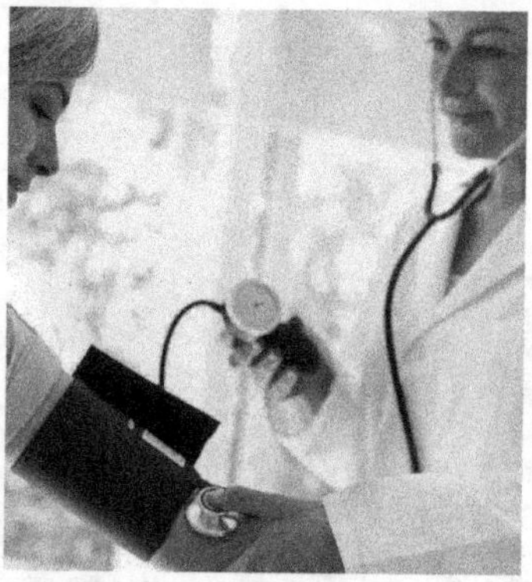

______ take BP

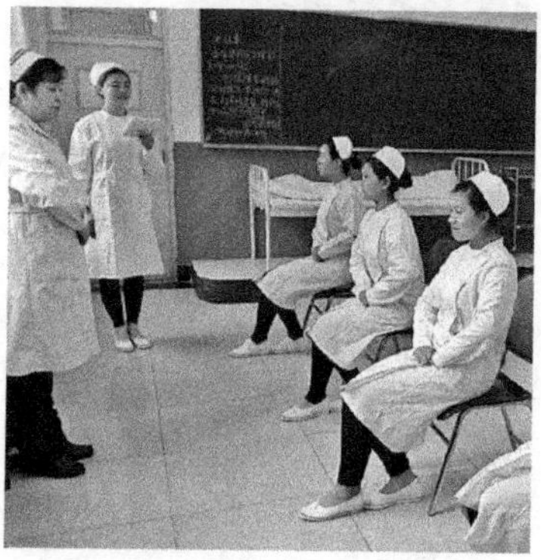

______ practice nursing etiquette

Ⅲ. Listen again and match the person with what they are doing now.

Mary	is taking BP.
Nancy	are having nursing practice class.
Nursing class 1	is giving an injection.
We	is practicing nursing etiquette.

Ⅳ. Look at the pictures. Make conversations.

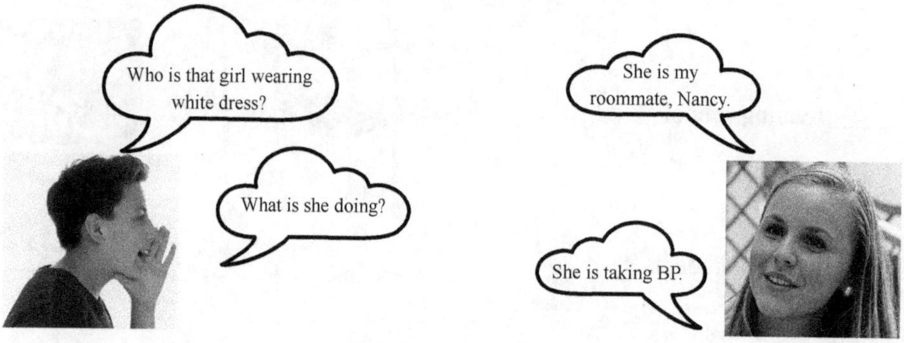
Who is that girl wearing white dress?
She is my roommate, Nancy.
What is she doing?
She is taking BP.

DIALOGUE

Role-play the conversation

Lily: Hello, Mary! Long time no see! How was your holiday?

Mary: Hi! Lily! I had a very busy holiday.

Lily: Really? Oh, Mary, this is Sarah, my roommate. Sarah, this is Mary, my middle school classmate.

Sarah: Nice to meet you, Mary! I'm from the United States. What about you?

Mary: Nice to meet you, too! I'm from Canada.

Sarah: Oh, I see. I major in Nursing and I'm in Nursing Class 1, and you?

Mary: My major is nursing, too. While I'm in Nursing Class 4.

Lily: We're going to the training room. Will you go with us?

Mary: Yes, certainly, let's go.

READING

Ⅰ. Read the passage and tell "How to become a qualified nurse".

My Aunt is Always Young

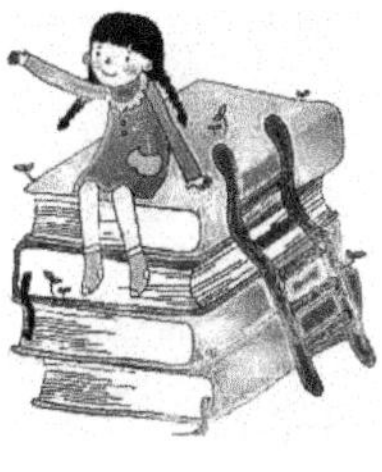

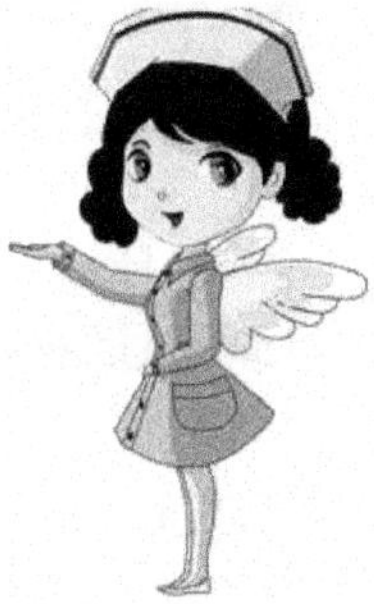

My aunt Jennifer is a head nurse. She is in Australia. She is working for a big hospital.

Being a nurse is her dream. After graduation from a junior middle school, she entered a nursing school and became a nursing student. During three years in the school, she studied nursing knowledge hard and drilled nursing skills diligently. While passing nursing qualification test, she graduated and became a registered nurse. She has been working in this big hospital for over 20 years.

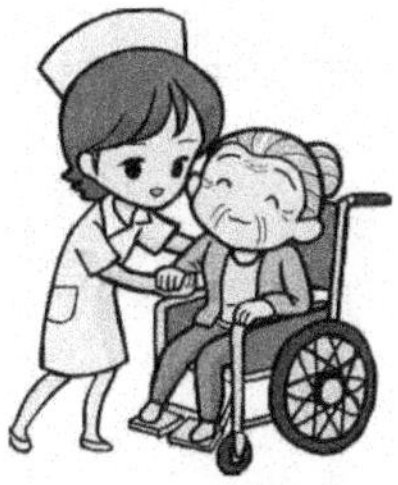

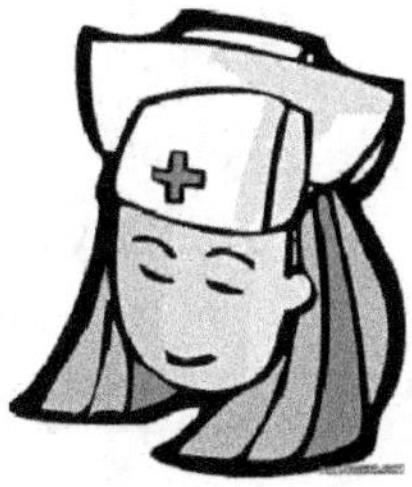

She must be at least forty years old. In spite of this, if anyone ever asks her how old she is, she always answers, "Darling, it must be terrible to be grown up!"

I am proud of my aunt.

Ⅱ. Find out your unknown words and phrases, written down and look up them.

Words	Meanings

Ⅲ. EXERCISES.

Reading Comprehension

1. The story about Jennifer suggests that ______

   A. My aunt is young. B. My aunt is old.

   C. My aunt is a qualified nurse. D. My aunt is a nursing teacher.

2. Which of the following statements is true?

   A. We know exactly how old Jennifer is.

   B. We don't know exactly how old Jennifer is.

   C. Jennifer is forty years old.

   D. Jennifer is over forty years old.

Structure

3. She must be at least forty years old, in my opinion, she ______ .

   A. has B. is C. can D. must

4. — ______ is she?

   — At least forty years old.

   A. How B. How big C. How many D. How old

5. She is working ______ a big hospital.

   A. in B. with C. by D. for

6. She graduated ______ a nursing school twenty years ago.

   A. in B. on C. by D. from

7. She has been working in this big hospital for over 20 years. It means "she has been working in this big hospital ______ ".

   A. 20 years B. less than 20 years

   C. more than 20 years D. unknown

Vocabulary

8. My aunt Jennifer is a head nurse. She is ______ .

   A. a nursing student B. a nursing teacher

   C. a nurse D. a nurse and a manager

9. She graduated from a junior middle school.
A. a nursing school B. a high school
C. a college D. a junior secondary school
10. She graduated and became a registered nurse.
A. young B. junior C. foreign D. enrolled
11. She is grown up. She is ______ .
A. very B. an adolescent C. a teenager D. an adult

GRAMMAR FOCUS

1. —Hello, Mary! Long time no see! How was your holiday?
—Hi! Lily! I had a very busy holiday.
2. —What is she doing?
—She is taking BP.
3. —Who is the boy using thermometer?
—He is my friend, Leo.
4. This is Sarah, my roommate. 这是我的室友萨拉。
5. What about you? 你呢?
e.g. I' m from the United States. What about you?
6. I major in... 我的专业是……
= My major is ...
e.g. I major in Nursing.
= My major is nursing.

Section B Extensive Reading

Ⅰ. Read the passage. Have you ever heard "The Lady with the Lamp"?

A Great Nurse—Nightingale

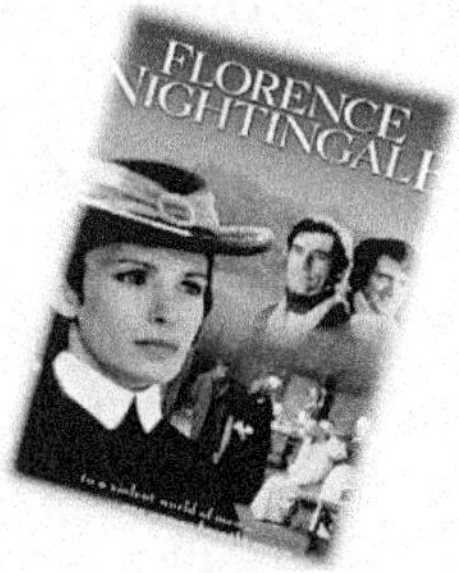

She could have lived an easy, comfortable life. But instead she chose to work hard and care for the sick. Florence Nightingale was one of the world's great nurses. Every year on her birthday, May 12, people celebrate International Nurses Day to remember the love and help that she gave to so many people.

Nightingale was born into a rich family in 1820 in Florence, Italy. When she was 24, she told her parents she wanted to be a nurse.

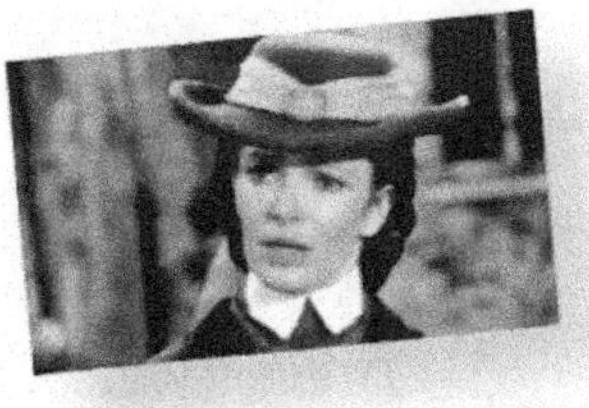

But they didn't like that idea. The family had lots of money, so they thought it would be better if she didn't work. Nurses were not well respected at the time. But Nightingale went on with her dream. She went to Germany to learn to be a nurse. There were no nursing schools at the time. She had to learn by practicing.

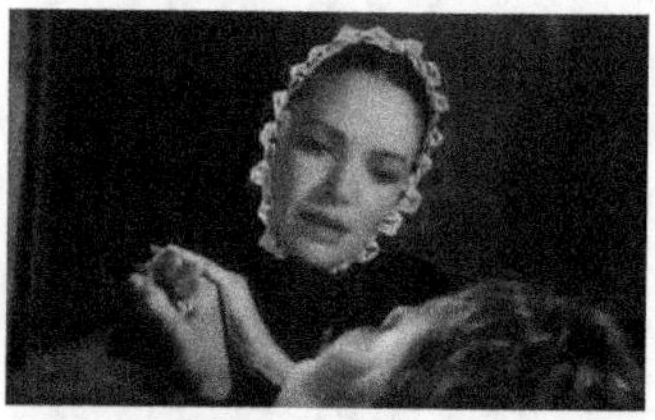

During a war in 1854, Nightingale and a team of 38 nurses from England went to care for soldiers near Turkey. She made the hospitals much cleaner there.

At night, she needed to look after the soldiers. She carried a lamp with her, and the soldiers began to call her "The Lady with the Lamp".

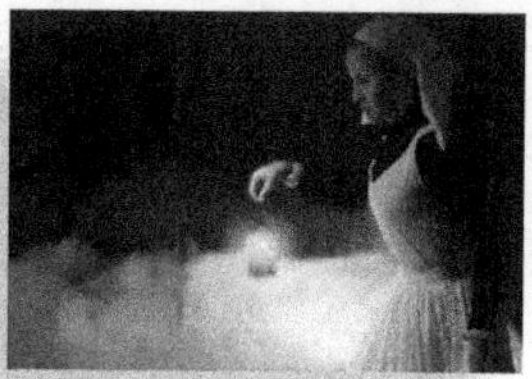

In 1860, after the war, Nightingale opened the first nursing school. She also worked to make hospitals better and make rules for nurses. She died in 1910 in London, England at age 90.

Nightingale's birthday became International Nurses Day in 1912.

Ⅱ. Find out your unknown words and phrases in the text, written down and look up them.

Words	Meanings

Ⅲ. According to the passage, fill T for true or F for false.

1. ______ Nightingale was born into a poor farmer family.
2. ______ Nightingale's parents supported her to be a nurse.
3. ______ Nightingale opened the first nursing school in the world.
4. ______ International Nurses Day, May 12th, is to celebrate the victory of the war.
5. ______ Florence Nightingale was one of the world's great nurses.

Ⅳ. Read, recite and sign.

Nightingale pledge

I solemnly pledge myself before God and in the presence of this assembly,
to pass my life in purity and to practice my profession faithfully.
I will abstain from whatever is deleterious and mischievous,
and will not take or knowingly administer any harmful drug.
I will do all in my power to maintain and elevate the standard of my profession,
and will hold in confidence all personal matters committed to my keeping and all family affairs coming to my knowledge in the practice of my calling.
With loyalty will I endeavor to aid the physician in his work,
and devote myself to the welfare of those committed to my care.

sign

南丁格尔誓言

余谨以至诚，
于上帝及会众面前宣誓：
终身纯洁，忠贞职守，
尽力提高护理标准；
勿为有损之事，
慎守病人家务之秘密，
竭诚协助医之诊治，
勿谋病者之福利。
谨誓！

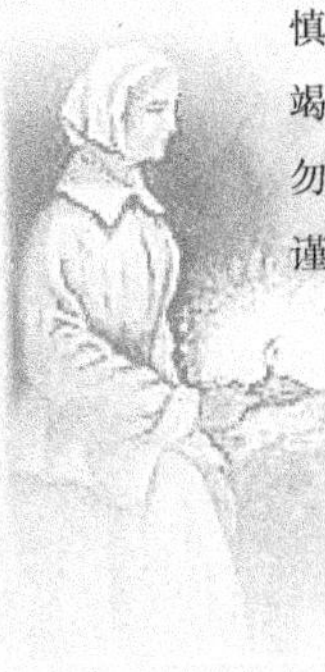

Section C *Writing*

Personal Data Form

在日常生活中，我们常常会填写一些包含个人信息的英文表格，如学生登记表、住宿登记表、考试报名表、申请表等。在这些表格中，我们需要提供一些相关的个人信息，如姓名、性别、年龄、出生日期、国籍、婚姻状况、家庭住址、电话、电子邮件地址等。

SAMPLE

The following is a part of a patient registration form. Please read and try to understand it.

Title: Ms.	First Name: July	Last Name: Smith
Nationality: American	Date of Birth:Nov. 12th,2001	
Address: No.17 Rush St., Chicago, Illinois U.S.A.60601		
Home Phone: (777)369-****	(777)369-****	
Mobile Phone:001-722-345-****	E-mail: July12@qq.com	

KNOWLEDGE

1. Title：称呼

常见的称呼有 Mr.（先生）、Mrs.（夫人）、Miss（小姐）和 Ms.（女士）等，以确定填表人的性别。对于女性，要注意三种称呼的区别。Miss 表示未婚女性，Mrs. 表示已婚女性，Ms. 适用于所有女性。

2. Name：姓名

其中 first name（give name）表示名；family name（surname/last name）表示姓，有些西方国家的人也有 middle name，即中间名。

3. Nationality：国籍

需要注意的是，在填写国籍的时候不能使用国家名，而应使用国家名的形容词形式。如中国国籍要用 Chinese，而不是 China。

4. Date of Birth：出生日期

英文的日期通常以月、日、年为顺序，月份可以缩写，日和年用逗号隔开。如：November 18th，2011 或者 Nov.18th，2011。

5. Address：家庭住址

英文地址的书写顺序与中文相反，应该遵循从小到大的顺序，即门牌号、街道名、区名、市（州 / 县）、国名、邮政编码。

EXERCISES

Fill in the following form with your own information.

Personal Data Form				
First name		Family name		Gender
Nationality		Date of Birth		
Family Address				
Telephone		Mobile Phone		
E-mail		ID/Passport Number		

Unit 2

Go to Hospital

Section A *What's the Matter with Mary?*

Language Goals: Talk about Health Condition.

WARM-UP

Ⅰ. Match the phrases with pictures.

________ an appalling headache

________ a high fever

________ a violent stomachache

________ a bad toothache

________ a terrible cough

________ a sore throat

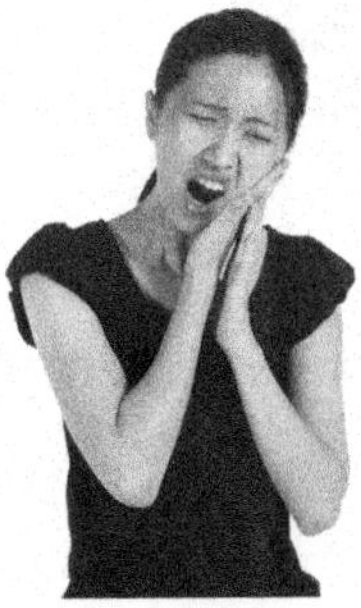

A

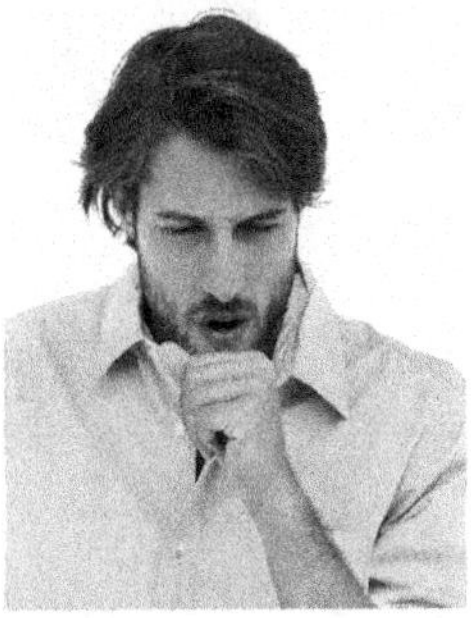

B

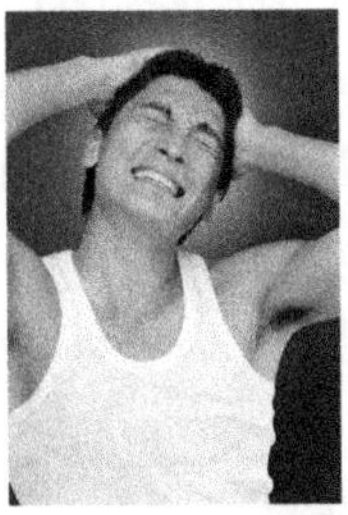

C

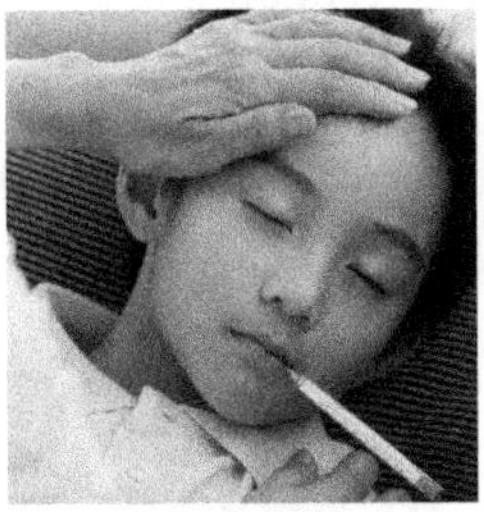

D

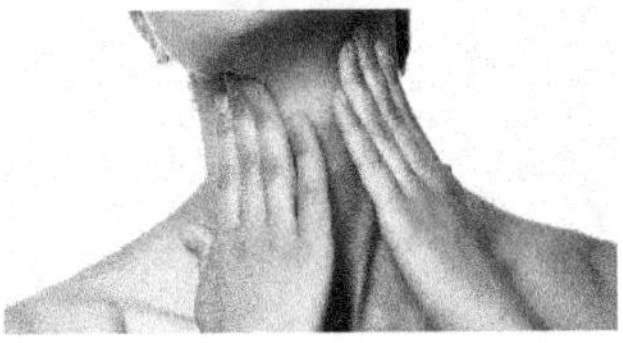

E

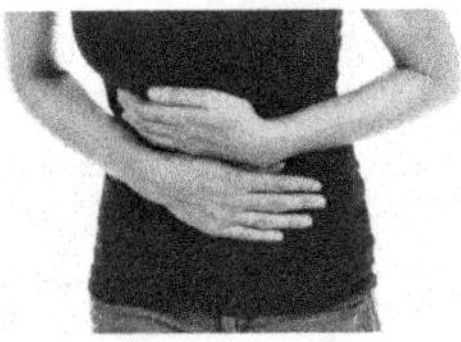

F

Ⅱ. Listen and number the pictures 1 to 4 in the order you hear them.

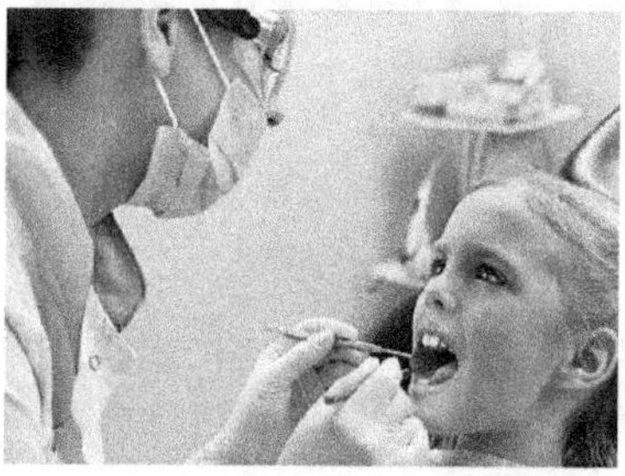

______ see a dentist

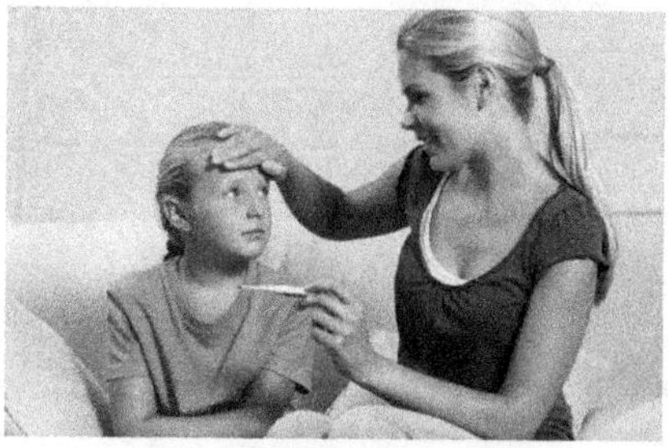

______ take one's temperature

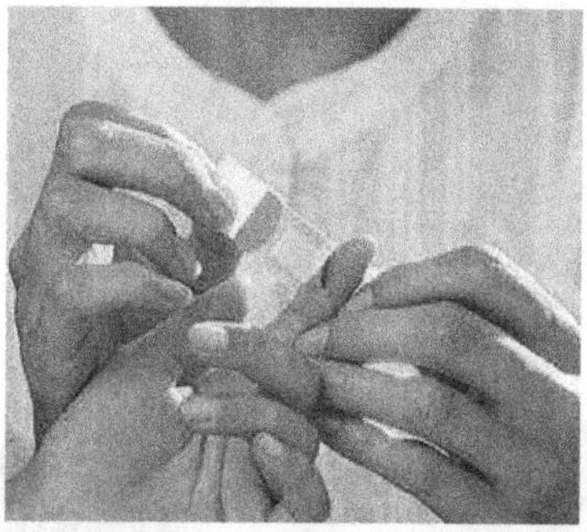

______ dress the wound

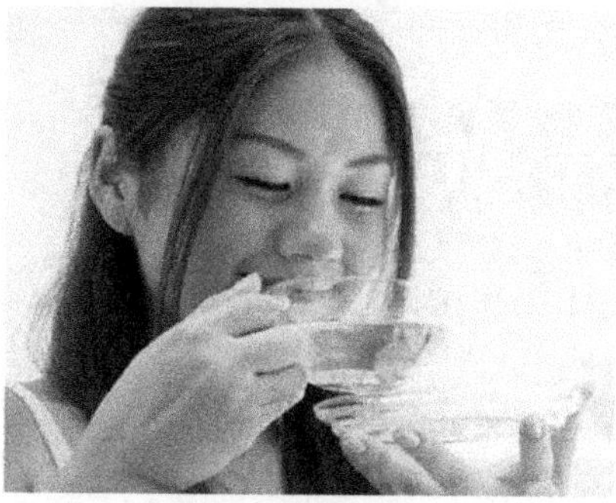

______ drink some hot tea with honey

Ⅲ. Listen again and match the symptom with what advice they should take.

toothache	drink some hot tea with honey
fever	see a dentist
cut myself	take your temperature
have a sore throat	put some medicine and dress the wound

Ⅳ. Look at the pictures. Make conversation.

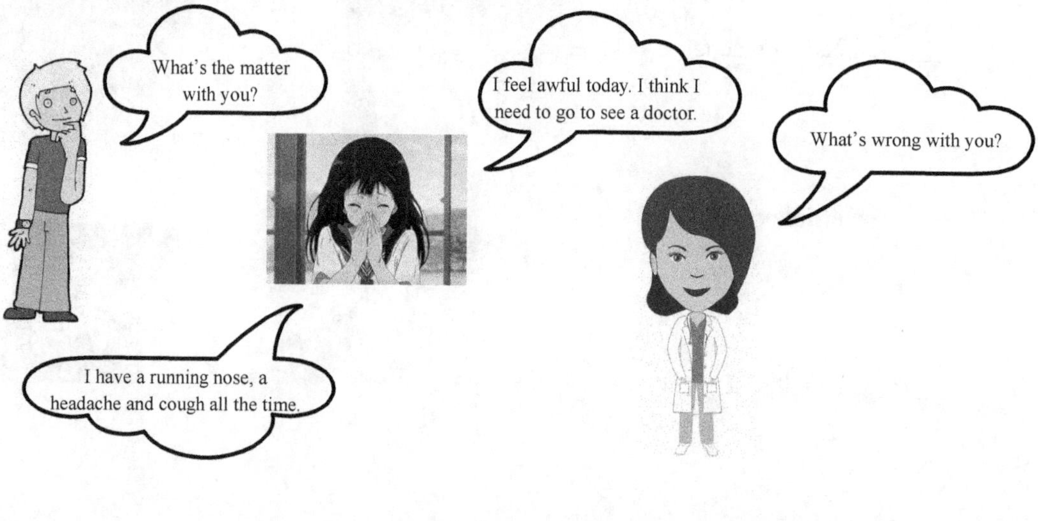
What's the matter with you?
I feel awful today. I think I need to go to see a doctor.
What's wrong with you?
I have a running nose, a headache and cough all the time.

DIALOGUE

Role-play the conversation.

Sherry: What's the matter with you?

Mary: My head feels very hot and I feel a little dizzy.

Sherry: OK, let me take your temperature.

Mary: I feel very cold, do I have a fever?

Sherry: Well, you have had a high fever.

Mary: Is it very serious?

Sherry: Don't worry. Take this medicine three times a day. You should drink more water and have a good rest.

Mary: Thank you.

READING

Ⅰ. Read the passage and tell "Doctor Sherry Brain's Busy Afternoon".

Doctor Sherry Brain's Busy Afternoon

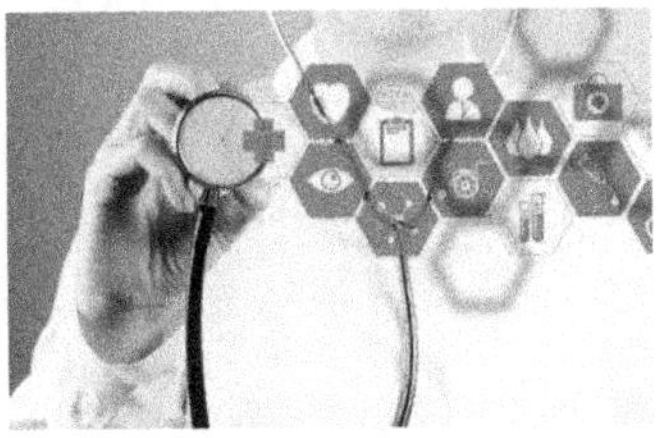

This afternoon, my friends and I visited the school clinic. Doctor Sherry Brain works at the school clinic.

The first one was Mary, who is in Nursing Class 4. It was a cold day, but she was in a very short skirt. She looked pale and kept coughing all the time. She told the doctor that she had a headache. After a careful check, Dr. Sherry told her that she had caught a cold and it was not serious. Dr. Sherry advised that she should take the pills three times a day for 3 days and remember to wear warmer clothes on cold days.

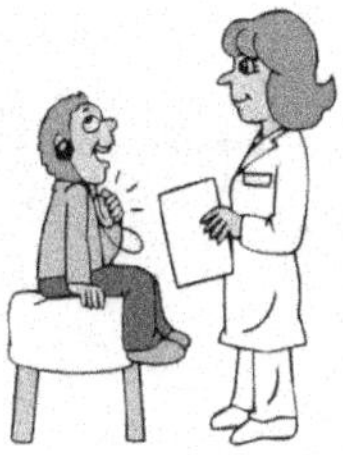

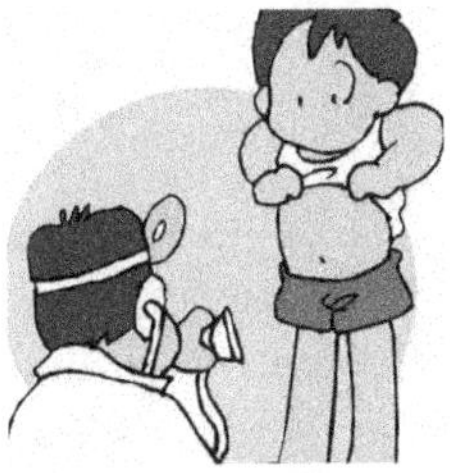

Sara, my roommate, was the second. She said that she had a stomachache. Dr. Sherry asked what she had for lunch. Sara said that she had 4 big hamburgers, a large Coca-Cola with ice as well as a large box of ice-cream. Dr. Sherry said, "What a huge lunch! Well, it is nothing serious. Just remember to exercise more and eat less!"

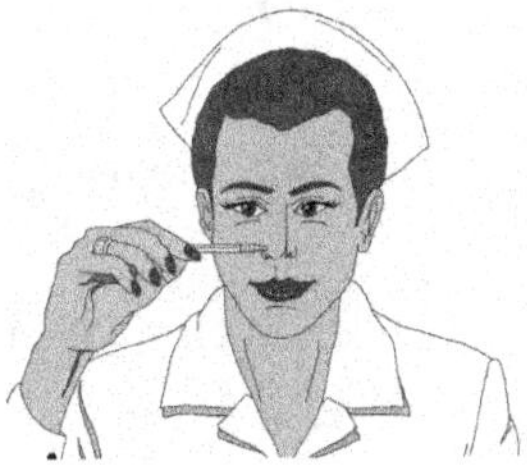

The last one was me. My name is Lily. I came to the clinic because I fell off my bike and hurt my right foot. Dr. Sherry asked me to lie down and put some ice on my right foot. After a while, I felt much better. Dr. Sherry told me to use ice on my right foot for 5 minutes each hour for the first 2 days when I went home. "Stay in bed for a week" , said Dr. Sherry.

What a busy afternoon!

Ⅱ. Find out your unknown words and phrases, written down and look up them.

Words	Meanings

Ⅲ. EXERCISES.

Reading Comprehension

1. Where did Mary, Sara and Lily go this afternoon?
   A. the school library　B. the school clinic
   C. the school canteen　D. the school playground
2. What's the matter with Mary?
   A. She kept coughing all the time and had a headache.
   B. She had a stomachache.
   C. She had a sore throat.
   D. She fell off her bike and hurt her right foot.

Structure

3. Dr. Sherry must have had a busy afternoon, she?
   A. must　B. haven't　C. isn't　D. didn't
4. — ______ the matter with Lily?
   — She fell off her bike and hurt her right foot.
   A. What　B. How　C. What's　D. Why
5. Doctor Sherry works ______ the school clinic.
   A. on　B. at　C. by　D. away
6. Doctor Sherry told Lily to use ice ______ her right foot for 5 minutes each hour for the first 2 days when she went home.
   A. on　B. to　C. besides　D. off
7. Dr. Sherry advised Lily to stay ______ bed for a week.
   A. to　B. off　C. in　D. away

Vocabulary

8. Mary looked pale and kept coughing all the time when she visited the school clinic. She was ______ .

A. wearing the white skirt
B. sick and uncomfortable
C. happy
D. busy

9. "After a careful check, Dr. Sherry told Mary that she had caught a cold." Compared with the following sentences, which one has the same meaning as "a careful check" in the story?

A. We arrived at the airport, checked our baggage and wandered around the gift shops.
B. They packed and checked out of the hotel.
C. Then you need a full body check.
D. I'll ring the hotel. I'll tell them we'll check in tomorrow.

10. Sara said that she had 4 big hamburgers, a large Coca-Cola with ice as well as a large box of ice-cream. Which one can replace "as well as" in this sentence?

A. to
B. by the way
C. which
D. and

11. Dr. Sherry told Mary that she had caught a cold and it was not serious. What happened to Mary? Which one is NOT the symptom of Mary?

A. She had a sore throat.
B. She got a cold.
C. She had a cold.
D. She caught a chill.

GRAMMAR FOCUS

1. — What's the matter with you?
— My head feels very hot and I feel a little dizzy.

① What's the matter with you? /What's wrong with you? /What are the symptoms? /What brings you here? 您哪儿不舒服？

② feel 表示"感觉"，属感官动词，可直接接形容词。feel very hot(感觉很烫)；feel a little dizzy(觉得有些晕头转向)。

2. Let me take your temperature. 让我给你测量下体温。

① let sb. do sth. 让某人做某事。

② take one's temperature 给某人测量体温。

3. have a fever 发烧；have/run a high fever 发高烧。

4. Take this medicine three times a day. 服用此药，一日三次。

e.g. Take a spoonful of this medicine three times a day after meals. 这药一天服三次，每次服一汤匙，饭后服用。

5. You should drink more water and have a good rest. 你应该多喝水，并且好好休息。

Section B Extensive Reading

Ⅰ. Read the passage. Have you ever got to know "Hospitals"?

Hospitals

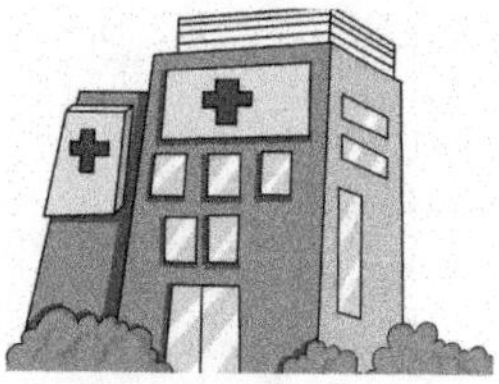

Hospitals are the places for the treatment and care of people who are ill or sick or who need a doctor, for example, in pregnancy. They may also be the center for medical research and the training schools for doctors, nurses, and other medical workers.

Hospitals may be divided into general hospitals and special hospitals. The general hospitals have many different departments: medical, surgical, pediatric, obstetric, gynecological, dental and traditional medicine. Patients of all ages and with different illnesses and injuries can be treated in the general hospitals. Other hospitals provide more specialized care. For example, some hospitals treat patients with chronic illnesses and offer facilities for long-term care. Others take patients of only one age group, such as children, or patients with one particular illness, such as tuberculosis.

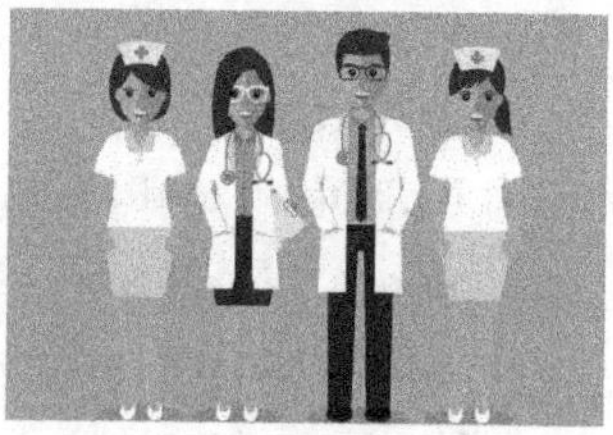

A hospital mainly consists of two major departments: the out-patient department and the in-patient department. There is also an emergency room. There are consulting rooms in the out-patient department. And there are wards and intensive care units in the in-patient department. Wards may be divided into various kinds, such as medical, surgical, maternity, isolation and observation wards. Each ward has several hospital beds.

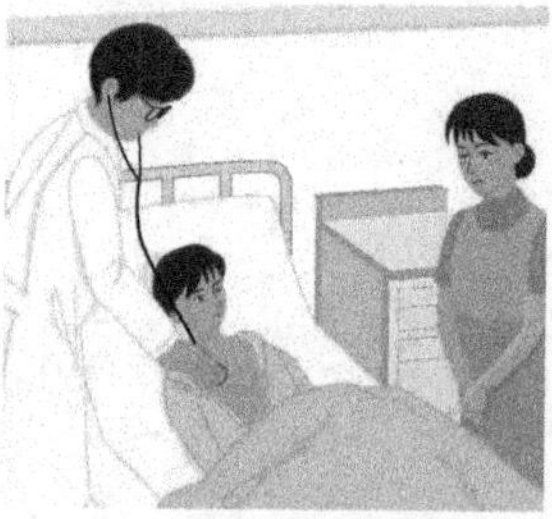

Doctors, nurses and other medical workers make up the staff of a hospital. Doctors, according to their specialties may be divided into physicians, surgeons, eye-doctors, ear-nose-throat doctors, dentist, etc. Both doctors and nurses care for the patients. With doctors, however, the science of medicine comes first; with nurses, the art of healing comes first. People say: Doctors treat diseases; nurses treat patients. Hospital patients may see their doctors only for a few minutes each day. But they see nurses much more, because nurses provide most of hospital patient care. They watch over the patient 24 hours a day.

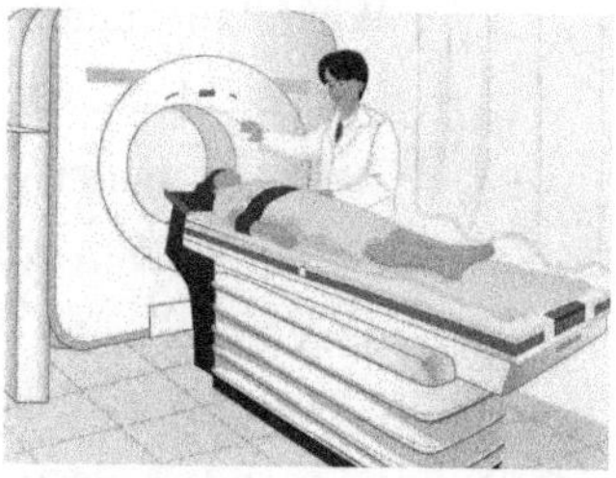

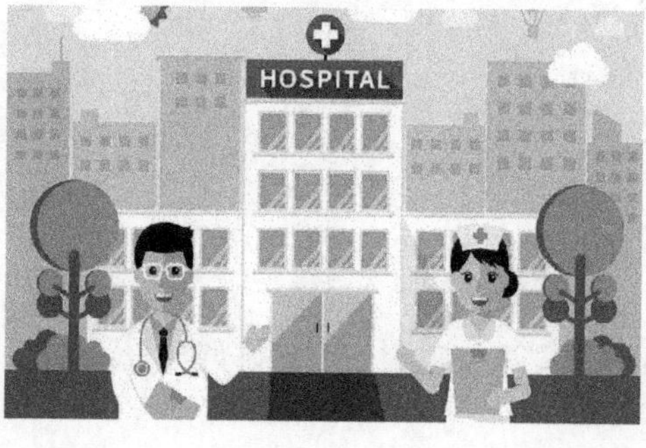

Ⅱ. Find out your unknown words and phrases in the text, written down and look up them.

Words	Meanings

Ⅲ. According to the passage, fill T for true or F for false.

1. ______ Hospitals are the places for the treatment and care of animals which are ill or sick or who need a doctor, for example, in pregnancy.
2. ______ Hospitals may be divided into general hospitals and special hospitals.
3. ______ Patients of all ages and with different illnesses and injuries can be treated in the special hospitals.
4. ______ A hospital mainly consists of two major departments: the out-patient department and the in-patient department.
5. ______ Hospital patients may see their nurses only for a few minutes each day. But they see doctors much more, because doctors provide most of hospital patient care.

Section C Writing

Notice

英语中的 Notice 包括告示、启示、通知等，目的是告诉公众某件事情或某项活动。如关于会议、讲座或某项活动的简单通知以及关于单位或组织的一些政策、措施和安排等。内容上明确简洁，一般包括事由、时间、地点以及涉及的人（四个 W，即 what, when, where, who）。

SAMPLE

The following is a seminar notice. Please read and try to understand it.

Seminar

"Safe Medication"
Thursday, 15th November
From 9:00am to 11:00am
In the conference room
For more information, please contact 010-34521186
All are welcome

KNOWLEDGE

1. Date/time：发出通知的日期

如果有发出通知的日期，按照月、日、年的顺序写在题目的右上角处。

2. Subject/Name : 题目

通常以 Notice 或 NOTICE 为题目，或者是以 Seminar（研讨会）、Speech(讲座）等活动、会议为题目。写在通知正文上方的正中央。

3. Activity：活动（演讲、比赛、会议、聚会等）具体内容

活动、演讲、会议等主题内容往往直接跟在题目的下一行。

4. Specific time：活动、会议、讲座等通知的具体时间

英文的日期通常以月、日、年为顺序，月份可以缩写，日和年用逗号隔开。常用结构：in June, 2017（2017 年 6 月 ）、on July 21st，2017（2017 年 7 月 21 日 ）、on Thursday, August 17th，2017（2017 年 8 月 17 日星期四）、at 7:00 pm on September 4th，2017（2017 年 9 月 4 日晚上 7 点钟）。

5. Place：活动、会议、讲座等通知的具体地点

英文地址的书写顺序与中文相反，应该遵循从小到大的顺序；活动、会议、讲座等经常出现的地点表达用语如：in Room 8, in the meeting room, in the stadium, in the conference room, in the teachers' office, in the lab, at the Friendship Theater, at the lecture hall 等。

6. Name of the issuing agency：发出通知的单位名称

如果有发出通知的部门、单位名称等，需要写在正文下方靠右下角处。

EXERCISES

Exercise A

Write a lecture notice according to the information given in Chinese. Some parts of it have been done for you.

1. ______________
（2017 年 10 月 20 日）

Notice

All the freshmen are required to attend the seminar
"2. ______________________". (“急救护理”)
Place: 3. ______________________（301 会议室）
Time: 4. ______________________（10 月 20 日周五下午 3 点）
5. ______________（护理学院）

Exercise B

Fill in the blanks with the information given in Chinese.

Speech

1. ______________________
（“如何提高你的英语口语”）
Speaker: 2. ______________（英语系教授 Amy Powell 女士）
Time: 3. ______________（9 月 18 日上午 10 点）
Place: 4. ______________（大礼堂）
For more information, please contact the
5. ______________（学生会）
All are welcome!

Unit 3

Treatment (Triage)

Section A *Where is the Registration Office?*

Language Goals: Talk about How to Ask and Give Direction in a Hospital.

WARM-UP

Ⅰ. Match the phrases with pictures.

________ Waiting Area

________ Information Desk

________ Examination Room

________ Emergency Dept.

________ Pharmacy

________ Registration Office

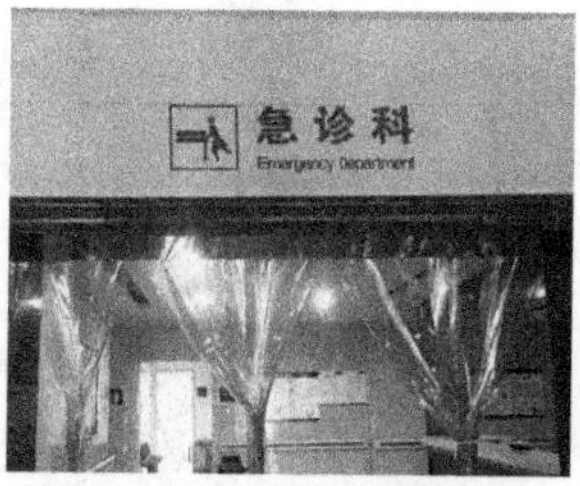

A

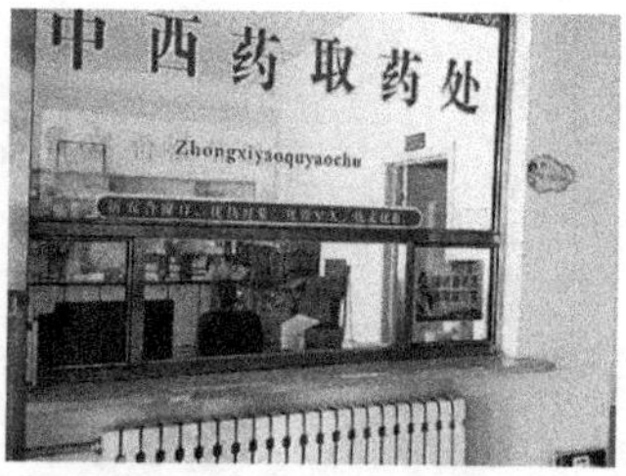

B

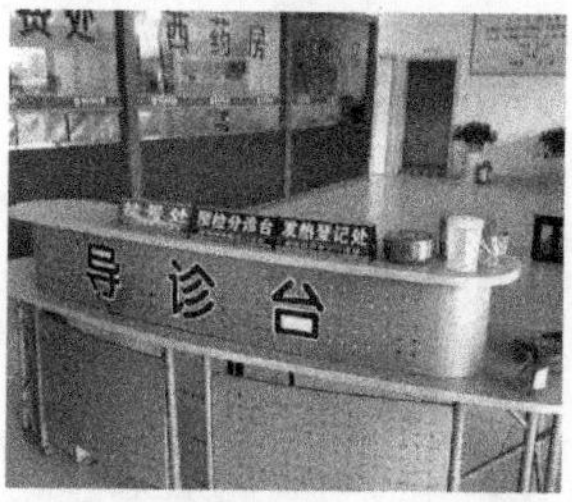

C

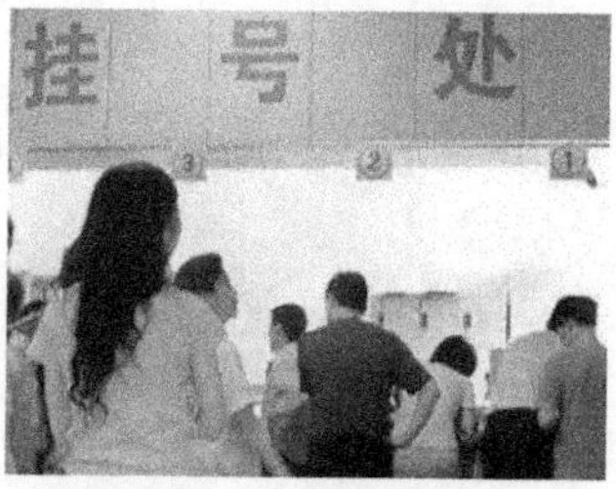

D

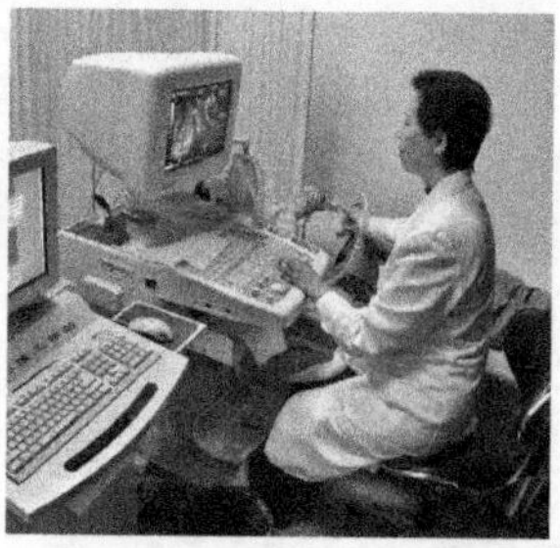

E

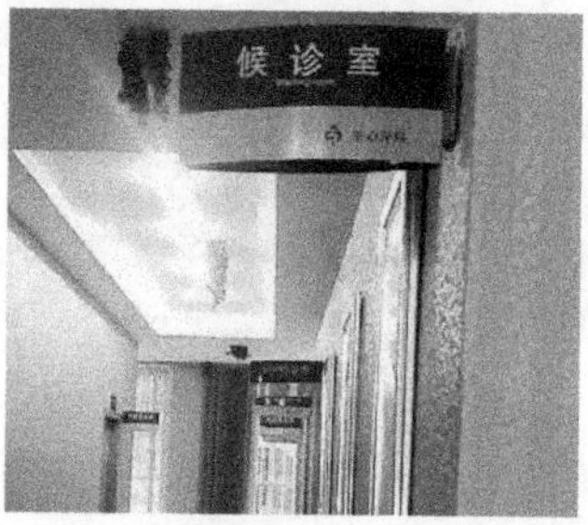

F

Ⅱ. Listen and number the pictures 1 to 4 in the order you hear them.

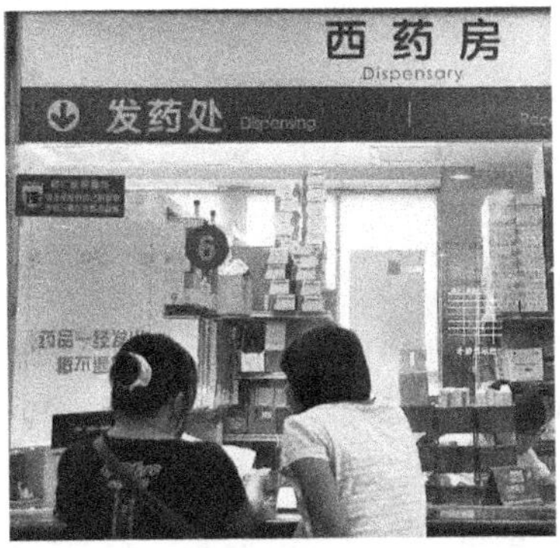

___get the medicine

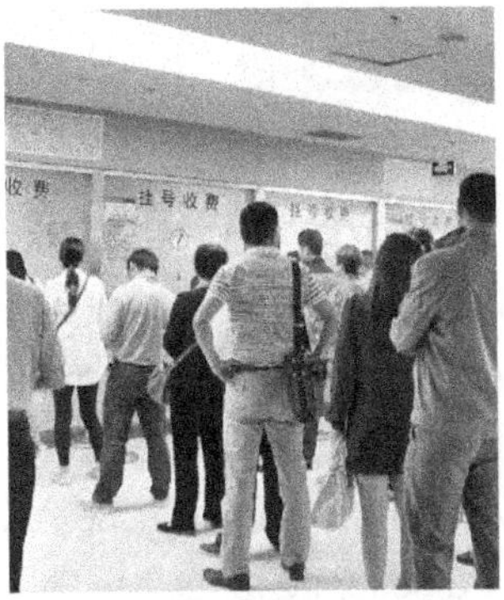

___queue for registration

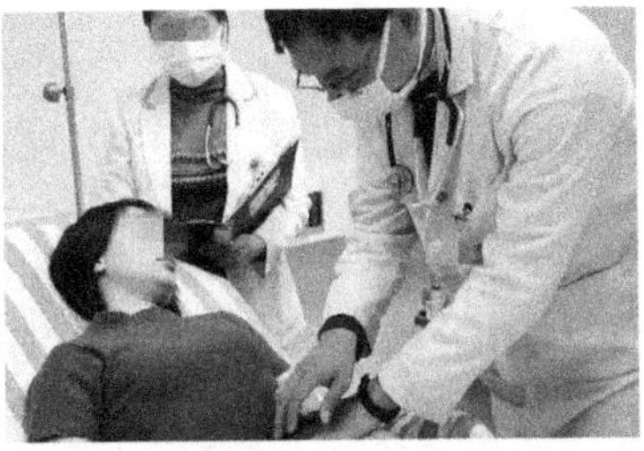

___examine the patient

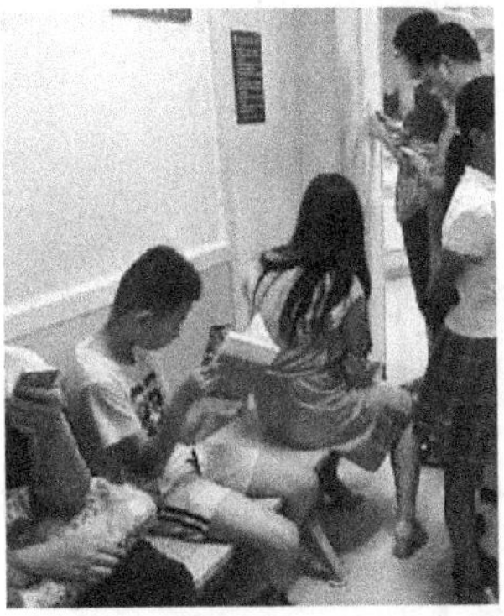

___wait to see the doctor

Ⅲ. Listen again and match the people with what and where they are doing.

queue for registration	at the pharmacy at the corner.
get the medicine	outside the Medical Department.
wait to see the doctor	in the examination room on the second floor.
examine the patient	at the lobby on the first floor.

Ⅳ. Look at the pictures. Make conversations.

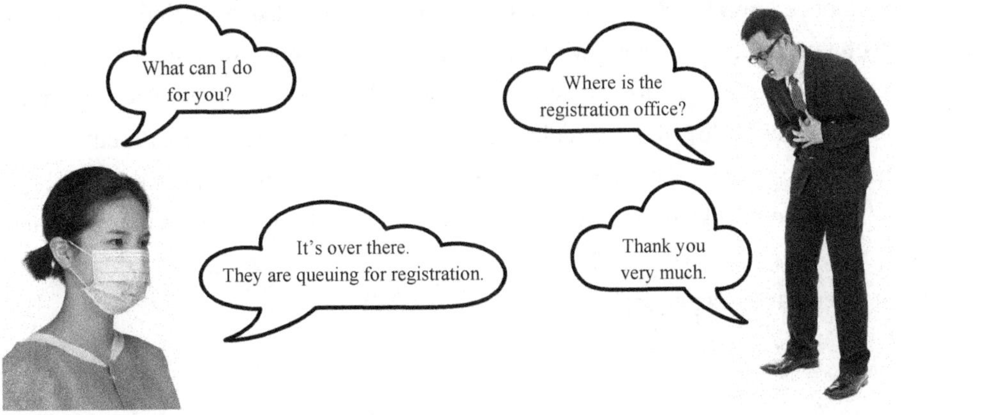

DIALOGUE

Role-play the conversation.

Nurse: Good morning, sir. What can I do for you?

Patient: Excuse me, Miss. Where is the registration office, please?

Nurse: Follow me, please. Look at that line over there. They are queuing for registration.

Patient: I have a little stomachache. Which department should I register?

Nurse: You'd better go to the Medical Department.

Patient: Fine. But can you tell me how to get to the Medical Department, please?

Nurse: Take the lift to the third floor and then go along until you see the sign on your right.

Patient: Thank you very much.

Nurse: You are welcome.

READING

Ⅰ. Read the passage and tell "Which floor is the Medical Department on? "

What an Embarrassing Experience!

My name is Sam. I'm a businessman from America. Last summer, I had to travel to London for five days because of my work. Maybe I was too tired and had a cold, so on my second day in London, I had got a high fever. In order not to influence the next work, I went to a local general hospital for medical treatment immediately.

After I got to the hospital, the triage nurse told me that I should register Medical Department, and told me it was on the third floor, the right hand side at the end. So I took the elevator to the third floor at once, went straight to the end. Because of a headache, I lined up without looking at the department sign. But, after a while, I felt something wrong. Why the queue was full of females? I looked up at the department sign. Oh, my God, it was Gynecological Department. When I was at a loss what to do, the gynecologist told me: "The Medical Department is on the upper floor, young man, it's just above the room." I couldn't help asking, "Isn't this the third floor? " At that moment the people around me began to laugh, one of them said to me, "You must not be British."

What an embarrassing experience!

Ⅱ. Find out your unknown words and phrases, written down and look up them.

Words	Meanings

Ⅲ. EXERCISES.

Reading Comprehension

1. According to the passage, Sam comes from ______ .
   A. China B. UK C. US D. London
2. Which of the following statements is right?
   A. Sam went to London for traveling.
   B. Sam is male.
   C. Sam registered Gynecology Department.
   D. The triage nurse showed the wrong way to Sam.
3. For Americans, which floor is the Medical Department on?
   A. 1st B. 2nd C. 3rd D. 4th

Structure

4. The Medical Department is ______ the third floor.
   A. on B. in C. at D. of
5. The triage nurse told me that I should ______ the Medicine Department.
   A. to register B. register C. registering D. registered
6. I lined up without ______ at the department card.
   A. looking B. look C. to look D.looked
7. I couldn't help ______ , "Isn't this the third floor? "
   A. ask B. asked C. asking D. to ask

Vocabulary

8. In order not to influence the next work.
   A. finish B. do C. notice D. affect
9. I went to a local general hospital for medical treatment immediately.
   A. at once B. later C. in the future D. not now
10. The Medical Department is on the upper floor.
   A.under B. above C. next D. top

GRAMMAR FOCUS

1. — Where is the registration office?
   — Look at that line over there.
2. — Which department should I register?
   — You'd better go to the Medical Department.
3. — Can you tell me how to get to the Medical Department?
   — Take the lift to the third floor and then go along until you see the sign on your right.

英语中问路的句型有以下几种：

① Excuse me, where is... , please?
② Can/Could/Would you tell me the way to..., please?
③ How can I get to the...?
④ Could you tell me how to get to...?
⑤ Would you please show me the way to...?

你可以这样告诉别人路线：

① Go along/down the street/ road.
② Turn right/left at the... turning/ crossing.
   Taking the... turning on the left/right.
③ It's over there on the left/ right. It's near/beside/between...

Section B Extensive Reading

Ⅰ. Read the passage. Try to understand the word "Angels in White" .

Working Christmas Day

It was unusually quiet in the emergency room on December 25. I was triage nurse that day. I didn't think there would be any patients, sighing about having to work on Christmas. Just then five bodies showed up at my desk, a pale woman and four small children.

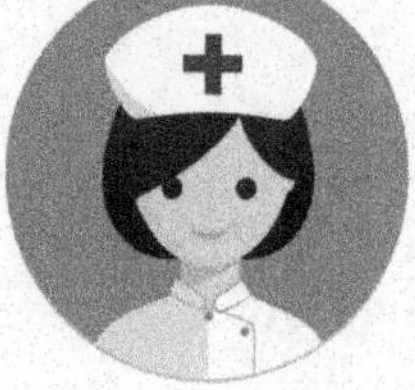

"Are you all sick? " I asked.

"Yes," she said weakly and lowered her head.

But when it came to descriptions of their presenting problems, things got a little uncertain. Two of the children had headaches, two children had earache, but only one could tell me which ear was affected. The mother complained of a cough but seemed to work to produce it.

Something was wrong, I didn't say anything but explained that it might be a little while before a doctor saw her. She responded, "Take your time，it's warm in here." Then, I checked their chart.

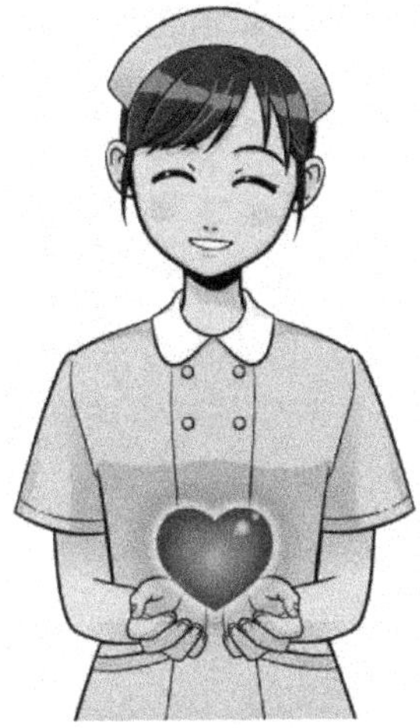

No address —— they were homeless. The waiting room was warm.

I went back to the nurses'station and mentioned we had a homeless family in the waiting room. The nurses, complaining of working on Christmas, turned to compassion for a family just trying to get warm on Christmas. The team went into action, much as we do when there's a medical emergency. But this was a Christmas emergency.

We were all offered a free meal on Christmas Day, so we took back that meal and prepared a big dinner for our Christmas guests.We needed presents. We collected from different departments candies, fruits and other things available that could be presents.As seriously as we met the physical needs of the patients, our team worked to meet the needs of a family who just wanted to be warm on Christmas.

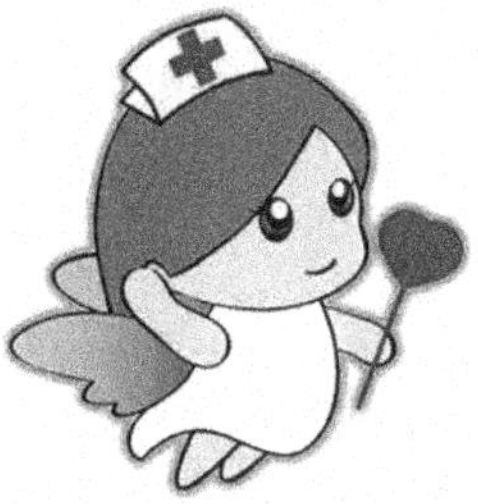

Later, as the family walked to the door to leave, the four-year-old boy came running back, gave me a hug and whispered, "Thanks for being our angels today."

Ⅱ. Find out your unknown words and phrases in the text, written down and look up them.

Words	Meanings

Ⅲ. According to the passage, fill T for true or F for false.

1. ______ The author was a triage nurse.
2. ______ There were four small children got sick on Christmas.
3. ______ The family were not homeless actually.
4. ______ The family got into the emergency room just because the emergency room was very warm.
5. ______ According to the passage, we can feel that Angels in White passed their love to the people in need.

Ⅳ. Nurses have four fundamental responsibilities:

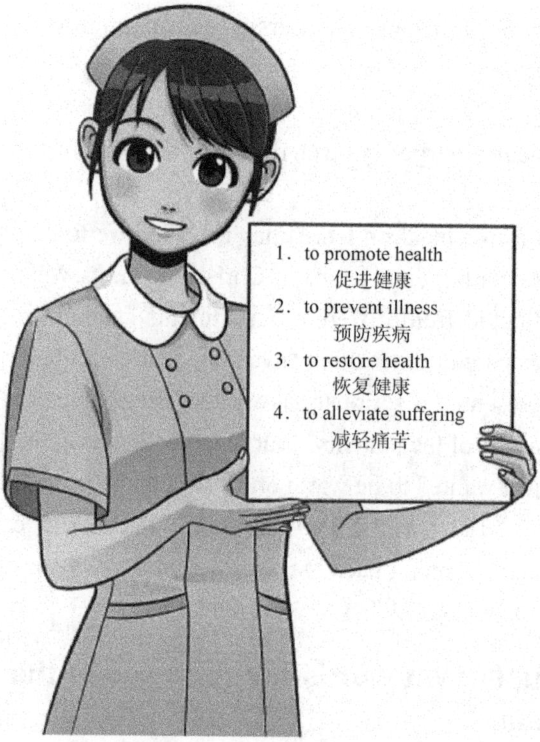
1. to promote health
促进健康
2. to prevent illness
预防疾病
3. to restore health
恢复健康
4. to alleviate suffering
减轻痛苦

Section C *Writing*

Plans

计划是在事情实际运作前人们所做的规划。一个好的计划不但能够帮助人们更好地实现既定目标，而且能够帮助人们高效合理地分配和使用有限的时间、金钱或资源。最简单的计划应包括两个部分，即时间（或钱数）和具体实施的内容。

SAMPLE

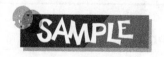

The following is a weekly plan of a head nurse. Please read and try to understand it.

Ms. Chen, a new head nurse in a general hospital, wants to finish the routine work better. Here is her weekly nursing plan.

Monday: Check and record the number of standing and first-aid drugs.（查对常备和急救药品数量并记录）

Tuesday: Clean the office.（打扫办公室卫生）

Wednesday: Tidy up the doctor' s orders, the injection forms and the nursing records.（整理医嘱单、注射单和护理单）

Thursday: Supplement the nursing station supplies.（补充护理办公室用品）

Friday: Sum up the total number of liquids.（总结液体总数）

KNOWLEDGE

1. 可简要介绍计划的背景，交代其依据。
2. 计划最重要的是时间、钱数安排和实施计划的步骤，按重要性和时间顺序，逐条列举。
3. 语言要简洁明了。

EXERCISES

Here is a plan for your internship. Fill in the following blanks according the meanings given.

In order to let student nurses to complete the internship task better and understand the practice goals, our hospital makes the following arrangements for the eight months' internship:

17th-23rd Jul. 2017 ________________（岗前培训）

24th Jul.- 23rd Aug. 2017 ________________（急诊科）

24th Aug.- 23rd Sept. 2017 ________________（内科）

24th Sept.- 23rd Oct. 2017 ________________（外科）

24th Oct.- 23rd Nov. 2017 ________________（妇科）

24th Nov.- 23rd Dec. 2017 ________________（儿科）

24th Dec. 2017 - 23rd Jan. 2018 ________________（骨科）

24th Jan.- 23rd Feb. 2018 ________________（中医科）

24th Feb.-16th Mar. 2018 ________________（手术室）

Unit 4

Giving Injections

Section A How Terrible the Injection is!

Language Goals: Talk about Giving Injections. Express Emotions.

WARM-UP

Ⅰ. Match the phrases with pictures.

________ syringe

________ injection

________ solution

________ IV infusion

________ needle

________ transfusion room

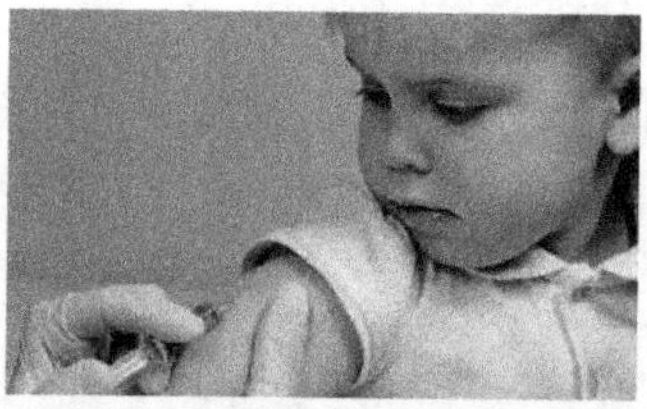

A

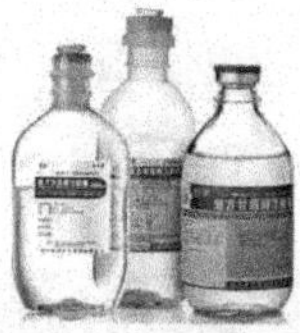

B

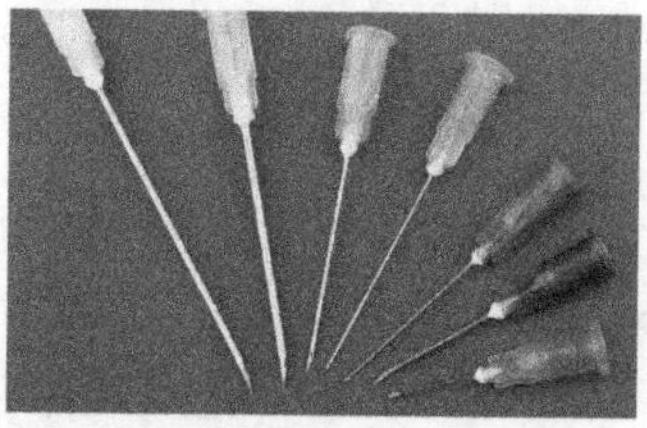

C

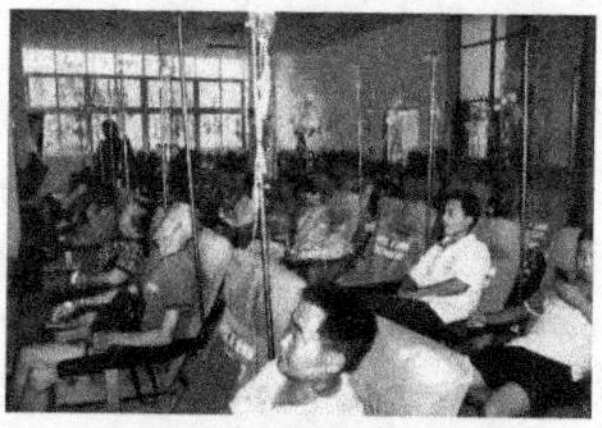

D

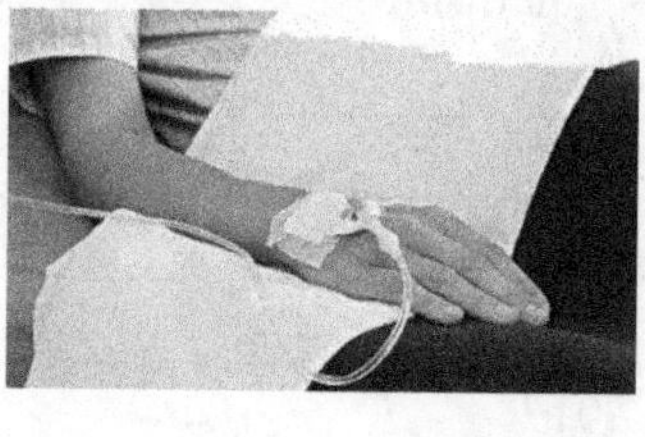

E

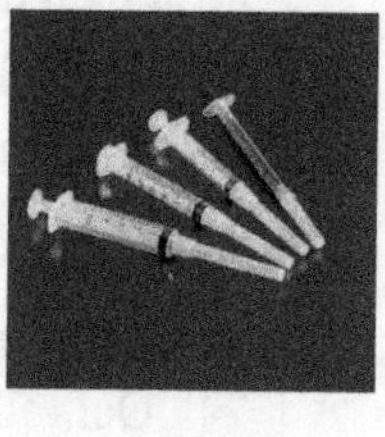

F

Ⅱ. Listen and number the pictures 1 to 4 in the order you hear them.

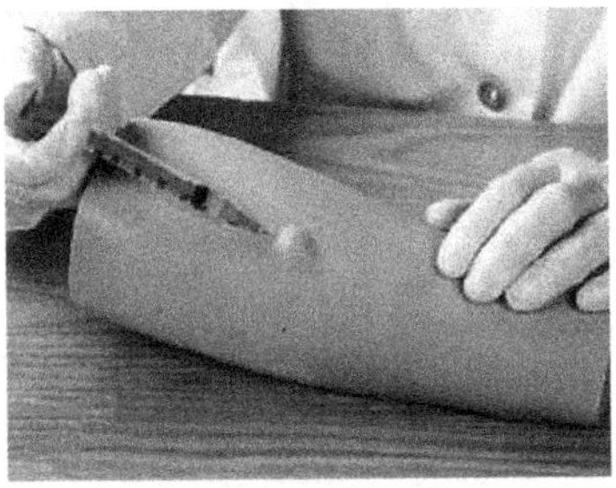

___ do a skin test.

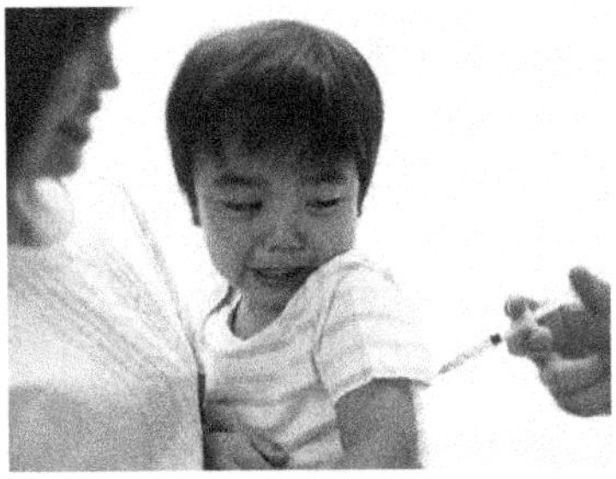

___ give an injection

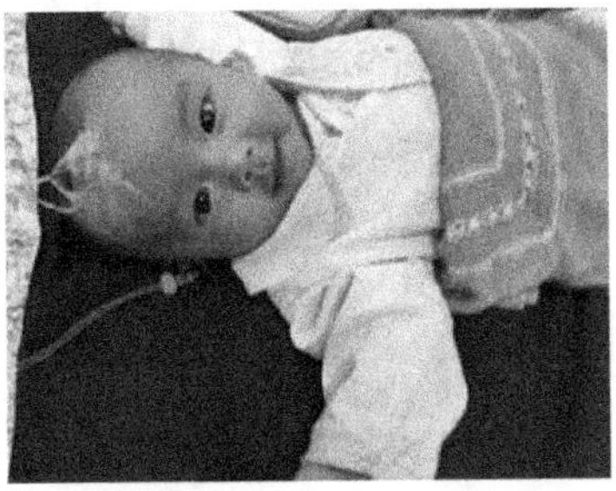

___ give IV fluids

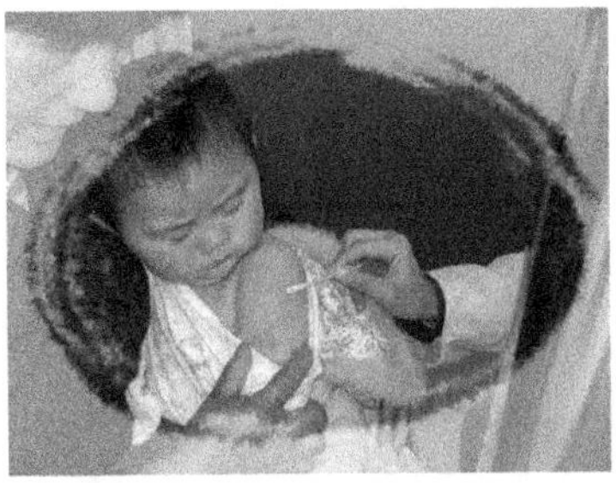

___ sterilize the skin

Ⅲ. Listen again and match emotions with the types of treatment.

is careful to	being sterilized his skin
is scared of	being given an injection
is curious about	do a skin test
is calm	give IV fluids

Ⅳ. Look at the pictures. Make conversations.

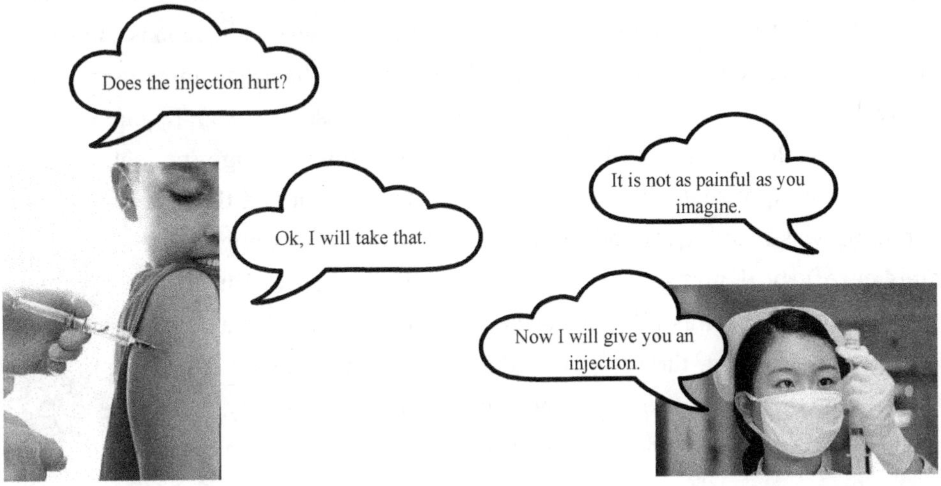
Does the injection hurt?
Ok, I will take that.
It is not as painful as you imagine.
Now I will give you an injection.

DIALOGUE

Role-play the conversation.

Mother: Excuse me, is this the injection room?
Nurse : Yes, please show me the prescription.
Mother: It is my daughter who is ill. Here you are.
Kid: I don't want an injection. How terrible it is!
Nurse : Hi, kid, don't worry. I'm sure you are brave. Besides, it will make you feel better soon.
Kid: Does it hurt?
Nurse: It is not as painful as you imagine. You will only feel a prick.
Kid: OK, I will take it.
Nurse: Is she allergic to any drugs?
Mother: No. How often should she have the injection?
Nurse: Twice a day. If there is anything wrong with her after the injection, please press the button, I will come soon. Kid, I will give you an injection now.

READING

Ⅰ. Read the passage and tell "How to serve patients better" .

My Experience Of Giving an Injection

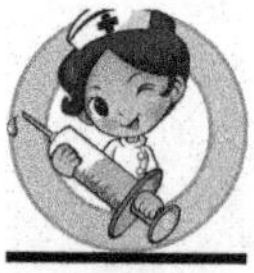

I have been working in the hospital as a practice nurse for one month. The head nurse asked me to give an injection for a patient this morning. I have given injections to my classmates at school, but this time was different—to serve a real patient! I was a little excited and nervous. When I was ill, I have been given several injections and some of them were painful. I wondered if I would cause pain when I inserted the needle through the skin. It is my duty to give the injection and it is good for the patient, so I must do as I am required.

At first I recalled the five rights which I would follow: the right patient, the right drug, the right dose, the right route and the right time. Then I examined the medicine to make sure that everything was ready. I wanted to be competent. After washing my hands carefully, I met my patient who needed a penicillin injection. I asked if she was allergic to the medicine, then I did a skin test. 20 minutes later, the result was that she was not allergic. After sterilizing her skin, I inserted the needle quickly and carefully. The patient was cooperative. I have done it!

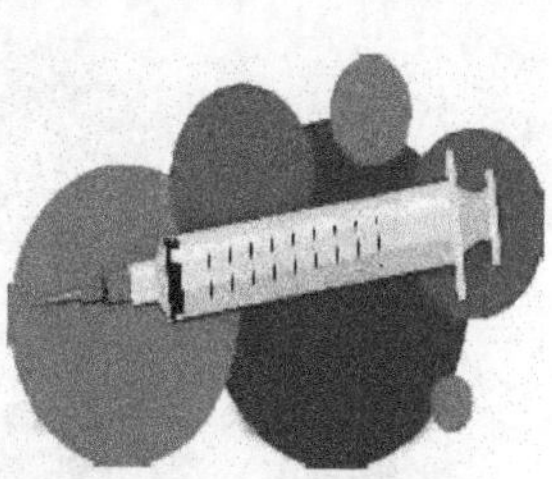

Ⅱ. Find out your unknown words and phrases, written down and look up them.

Words	Meanings

Ⅲ. EXERCISES.

Reading Comprehension

1. The story suggests that I am a ______ nurse.
   A. experienced B. inexperienced C. hard-working D. clever
2. Which of the following statements is true? ______
   A. I have never given shots to anyone before.
   B. As a patient, I was always given painless injections.
   C. I was sure that I would not cause pain.
   D. My injection today was a success.
3. Which one is not included in the five rights? ______
   A. the right patient and the right drug B. the right dose and the right time
   C. the right drug and the right route D. the right patient and the right place

Structure

4. It is my duty ______ give the injection and it is good ______ the patient.
   A. to, with B. to, of C. to, for D. of, for
5. The head nurse asked me ______ help a patient.
   A. for B. of C. by D. to
6. ______ a nurse, I have studied how to give injections at school.
   A. For B. As C. With D. To
7. After ______ the patient, I did a skin test for her.
   A. asked B. asks C. asking D. ask
8. Are you allergic ______ penicillin?
   A. to B. for C. of D. with

Vocabulary

9. I am a practice nurse.
   A. a home nurse B. a nurse's aid
   C. a student nurse D. a skilled nurse

10. I examined the medicine to make sure that everything was ready.
    A. act purposefully B. think about
    C. hope D. understand
11. I wanted to be competent.
    A. nice B. able to do my work
    C. clever D. hard-working
12. 20 minutes later, the result was that she was not allergic.
    A. before 20 minutes B. in 20 minutes
    C. after 20 minutes D. 20 minutes passing
13. I inserted the needle.
    A. pick up B. find
    C. give D. put something into the skin
14. The patient was cooperative.
    A. warm-hearted B. clever
    C. be willing to do as required D. do something with complaining
15. I have done it!
    A. I have given the injection successfully.
    B. I have helped the head nurse.
    C. I have finished the work on time.
    D. I have made the patient happy.

GRAMMAR FOCUS

1. –Do you know if you are allergic to it? 你清楚你是否对它过敏吗？
   –I have no idea. 不知道。
   – Now I will do a skin test to see, if you are allergic to it. 现在我要做皮试看你是否过敏。
2. –Is it painful? 疼吗？
   – A little. I believe you are brave, right? 有一点。我相信你是勇敢的，对吗？
3. Rest your arm on the table and relax. Hold still, please. 把胳膊放在桌上，放松。请保持不动。
4. Don't look at it if you are nervous. Now the needle is in. 如果你感到紧张，就不要看。现在我要打针了。

Section B Extensive Reading

Ⅰ. Read the passage. Do you know what IV infusions are?

Intravenous Infusions: Something to Know

Intravenous (IV) infusions are one of the most important treatments in hospitals nowadays. Both medical workers and patients should be cautious when using IV infusions.

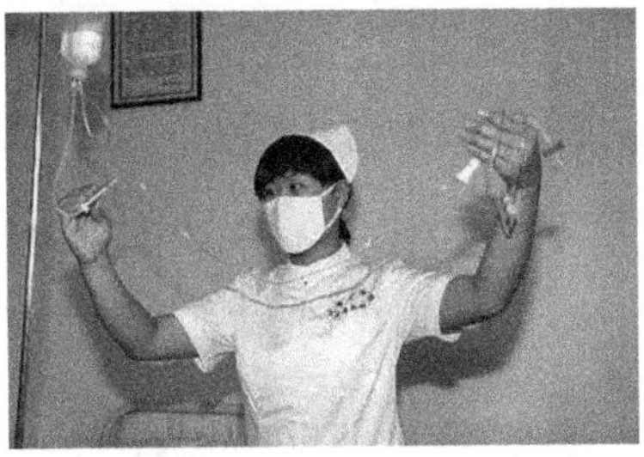

Introduction

Intravenous (IV) means "within vein" .

Intravenous infusions are commonly referred to as drips. The intravenous route is the fastest way to deliver fluids and medications throughout the body.

Usage

IV infusion of drugs is normally given to patients who cannot be treated orally or by injection. It can be used for fluid administration (such as correcting dehydration), to correct electrolyte imbalances, to deliver medications and for blood transfusions.

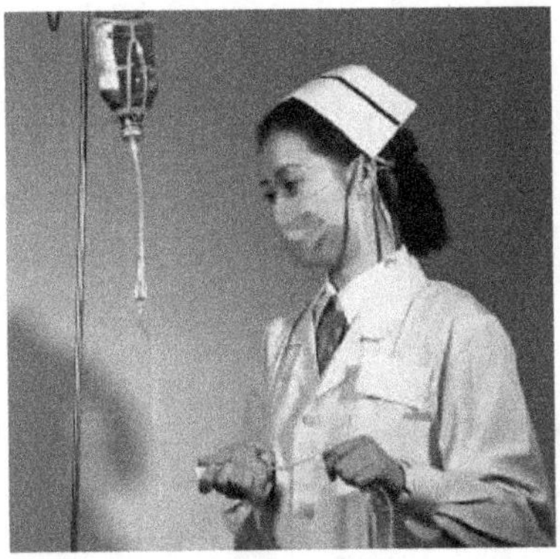

Site

The most common place for an IV infusion is in the hand. When the veins in the hand are unsuitable, the drip can be administered via vein in the arm.

Rate

In most cases, a patient receives medication at regular time until the IV bag is empty. The fluids cannot drip too quickly and must be given slowly in order not to overload the patient.

Side effects

While IV medication use is generally safe, it can cause mild or dangerous side effects. Medications given intravenously act on the body very quickly, so side effects, e.g. pain, infection, blood clots, allergic reactions, and other effects can happen fast. In most cases, a health care provider will observe you throughout your infusion and sometimes for a period afterward.

IV drug administration is a fast, effective way to send medication into your bloodstream, but every coin has two sides, so don't overuse it and if anything wrong happens, call your doctor or nurse right away.

Ⅱ. Find out your unknown words and phrases in the text, written down and look up them.

Words	Meanings

Ⅲ. According to the passage, fill T for true or F for false.

1. ______ IV infusions are the most important treatment.
2. ______ If a patient cannot take medicine orally, he can use IV infusions.
3. ______ The most common place for an IV infusion is in the arm.
4. ______ If a patient is in a hurry, the nurse can let the fluid drop more quickly.
5. ______ A patient is possible to be allergic to IV infusions.

Section C Writing

Personal Letters

作为一种特殊的文体和交流方式，私人信函是指与朋友、家人之间的往来书信，其内容比较自由，有固定的格式和构成，以下是五个构成部分：信头（含发信人地址、发信日期）、称呼（对收信人的尊称）、正文（发信人要说的内容）、结尾（发信人对收信人的谦称或致敬语）和签名（发信人姓名签字）。

SAMPLE

The following is a personal letter. Please read and try to understand it.

No.28 Changan Road
Ankang Health Company
Beijing, China
100060
October 16th, 20××

Dear Zhang Ming,

How time flies!

I'm not sure if you still remember me. I'm the woman who you met in the USA. At that time I told you I would be working in China.

I have been here for three months. I work at Ankang Health Company. I would love to visit you and your two friends, and also like to visit your university.

I look forward to hearing from you.

Yours,
Lucy Smith

KNOWLEDGE

1. Heading: 信头

完整的信头先写地址后写日期，地址的写法是从小到大，如 Sample 中的地址写法。在私人信函中，信头通常可以省略或者只写寄信日期。时间有英式与美式两种，例如：

英式：13th October, 2008

美式： October 13th, 2008

2. Salutation：称呼

称谓语用 Dear 称呼，如 Dear Zhang Lin，末尾用逗号。在信内地址下一两行处顶格写起，自成一行。

3. Body of letter：正文

正文是一封信的主体部分，通常在称呼的下一行写出。正文可采用齐头式或缩进式两种方法。

4. Complimentary close：结尾

结尾在正文之后一行的偏右方开始写，最后一个词后面用逗号。常用的结束语有：Yours/Yours sincerely/Yours truly/Yours faithfully...

5. Signature：签名
在结束语的下方签名。

EXERCISES

The following is a personal letter. Please fill it in with the Chinese information given below.

A letter to a doctor

September 15th, 20××

Dear Dr. Li,

I am writing to thank you and nurses for 1.______（照顾）______ me during the 2.______（手术）.Because of your careful 3.______（治疗）, I am able to 4.______（恢复）so quickly in a week. You are very 5.______（负责的）, so I just want to say thank you so much to all of you.

Best wishes.

Yours sincerely,

Wang Tian

Unit 5 Drug Treatment

Section A The Medicine is Wonderful.

Language Goals: Talk about Knowledge of Drugs. Give Medicine Instruction.

WARM-UP

Ⅰ. Match the phrases with pictures.

________ ointment

________ tablets

________ water aqua

________ oxygen mask

________ drug instruction

________ herbal medicine

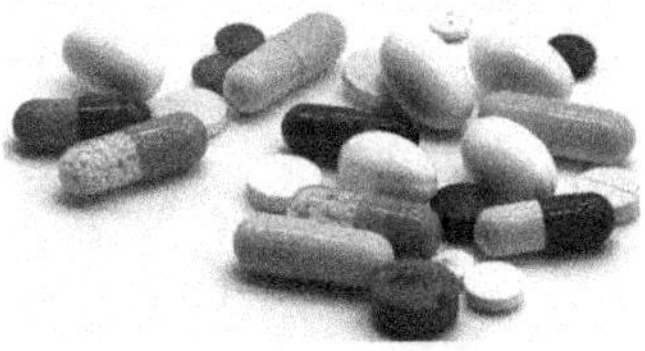

A

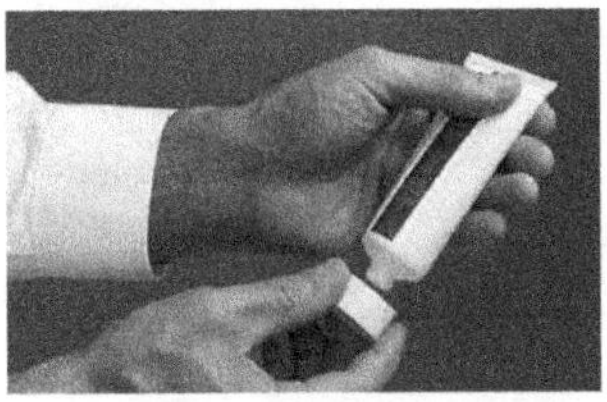

B

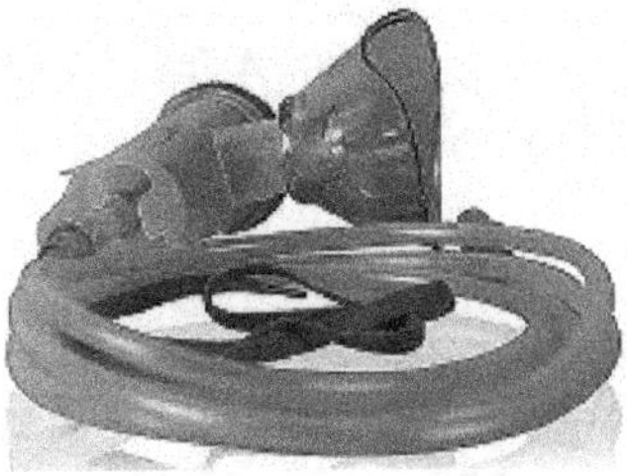

C

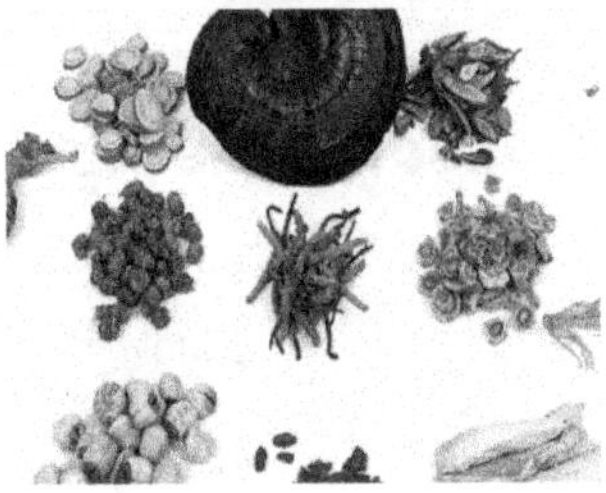

D

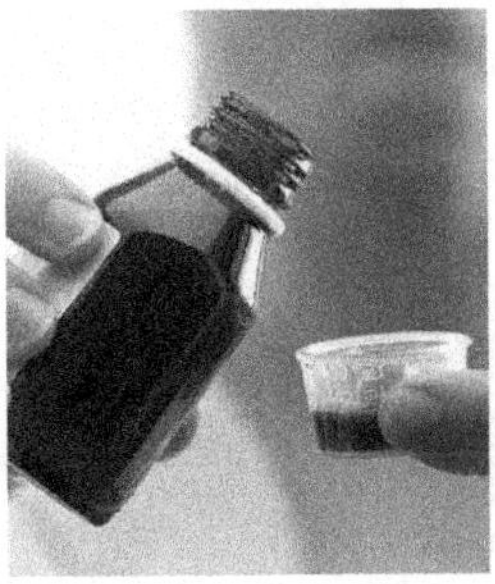

E

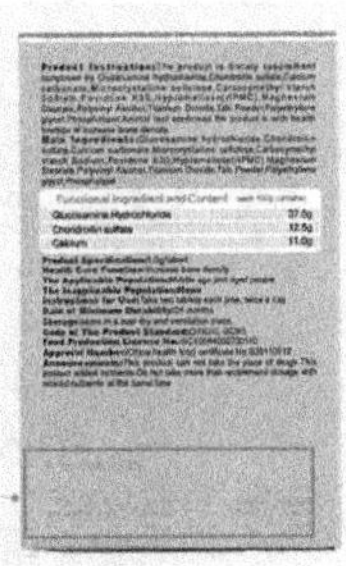

F

Ⅱ. Listen and number the pictures 1 to 4 in the order you hear them.

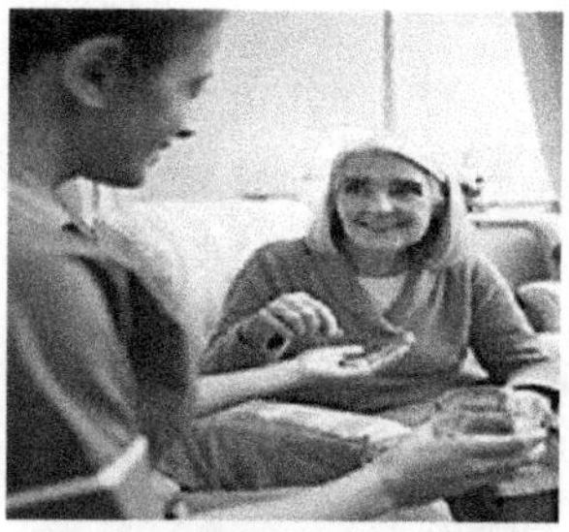

___ take western medicine

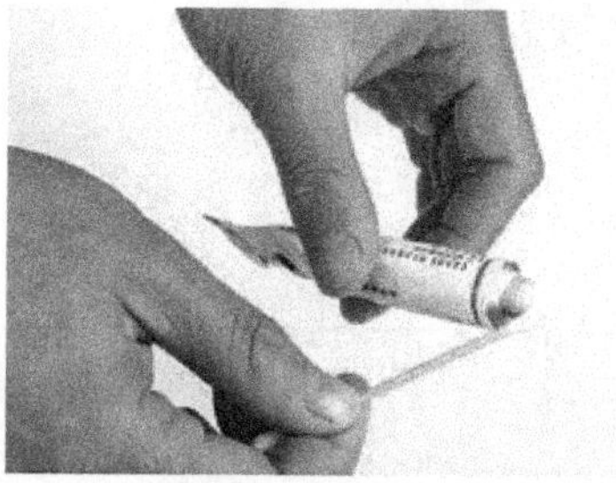

___ rub the ointment

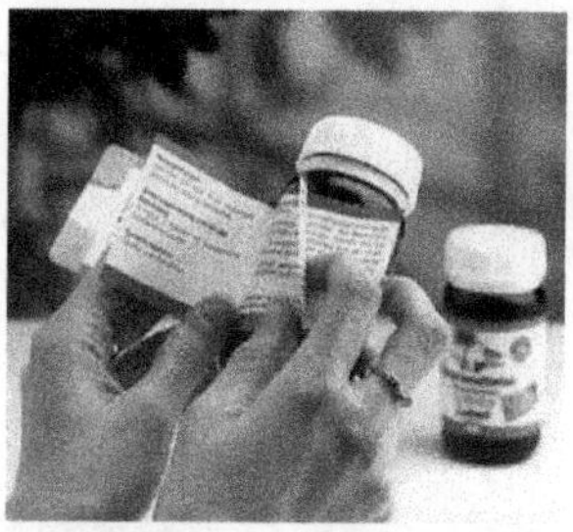

___ read the instruction

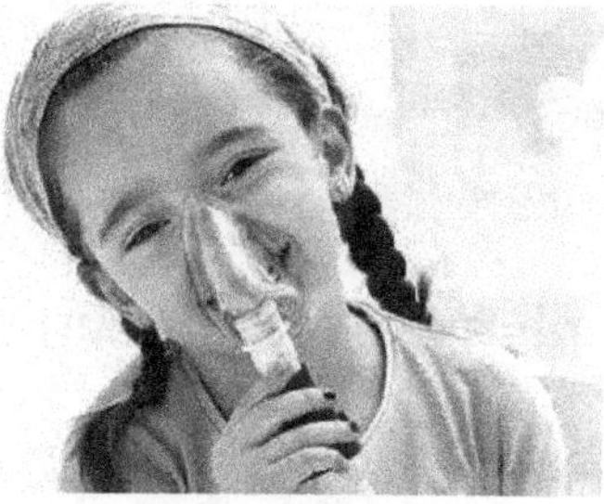

___ take in oxygen

Ⅲ. Listen again and match the medicine type with medication mode.

rub the ointment	before taking the medicine.
take western medicine	when she needs.
take in oxygen	two tablets three times a day on an empty stomach.
read the instruction	once a day at bedtime.

Ⅳ. Look at the pictures. Make conversations.

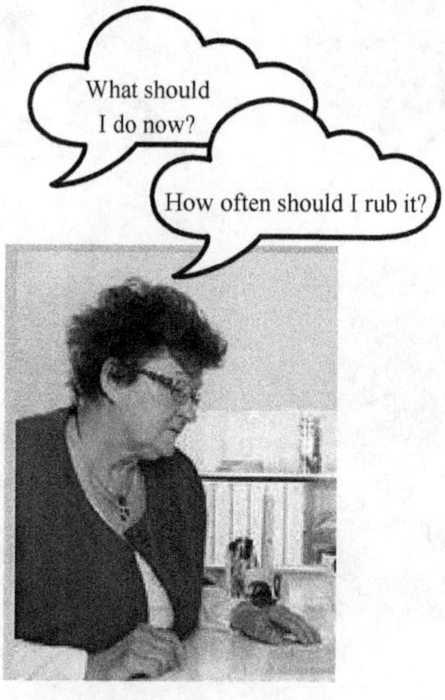
What should I do now?
How often should I rub it?

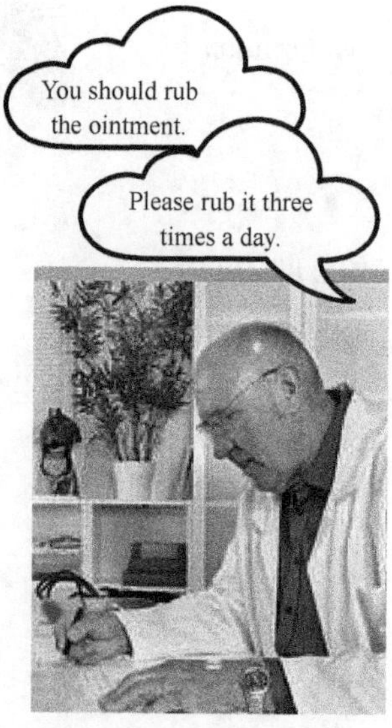
You should rub the ointment.
Please rub it three times a day.

DIALOGUE

Role-play the conversation.

Nurse: Good morning, Sir. Do you feel better?

Jack: Yes, I feel my knee is getting much better. The pain has almost gone. The medicine is wonderful!

Nurse: Great! Do you still keep taking Brufen?

Jack: Yes, 1 tablet each time, 3 times a day.

Nurse: Have you lost weight lately?

Jack: No, should I?

Nurse: Yes, you should lose weight to reduce the pressure on your joints.

Jack: OK. I'll do that. Thank you.

Nurse: You are welcome.

READING

Ⅰ. Read the passage and tell "Is there the medicine that can make us live forever?".

The Wonderful Medicine

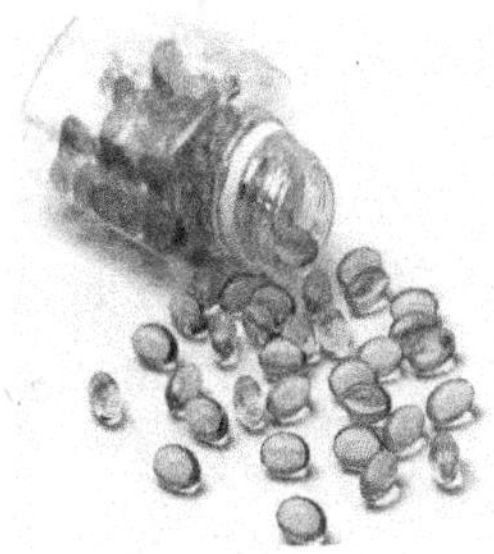

A man was selling medicine at a fair. At first, he sold bottles of a cure for colds for just a dollar a bottle.

Many people wanted to buy it and the man's young assistant collected money and handed out bottles of the cold cure.

Then, when he had a big crowd, the man held up a very small bottle. "And now, ladies and gentlemen," he shouted, "here is the medicine you have been waiting for. The cure for old age. Drink just one bottle of this and you will live forever."

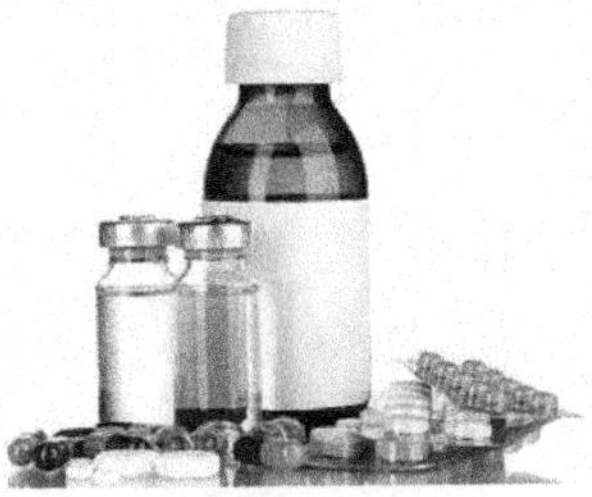

"And, ladies and gentlemen," the man continued, "I'm not going to charge you a hundred dollars a bottle for this wonderful medicine. No, ladies and gentlemen, I'm going to charge you just ten dollars a bottle. Think, my friends, for ten dollars you can live forever."

Most of the people in the crowed did not believe this.

One person shouted, "If it will make you live forever, why

don't you drink it? "

Another person cried, "Yes, you look as if you are at least sixty years old." "Thank you, sir, thank you," the man replied. "I'm so glad you said that. My real age is three hundred and twenty-nine."

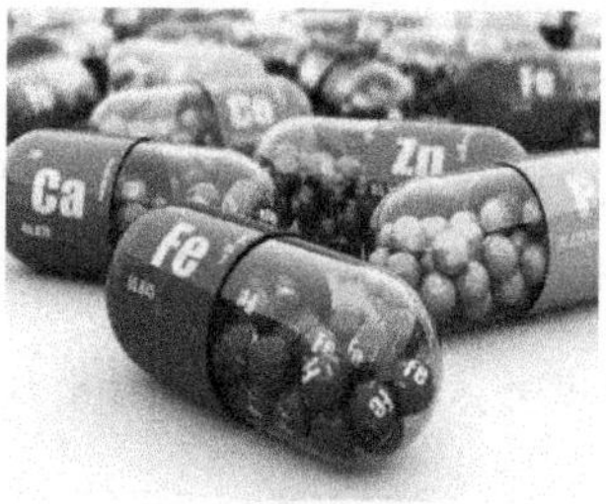

The crowd laughed at this, but there were still a few people who wanted to believe the man. One of them spoke to the man's assistant as she passed by. "Is that true? " he asked, "that he's three hundred and twenty-nine? "

"Don't ask me." the assistant said, "I've only worked for him for a hundred and fifty years."

Ⅱ. Find out your unknown words and phrases, written down and look up them.

Words	Meanings

Ⅲ. EXERCISES.

Reading Comprehension

1. Why didn't the people believe the man was selling medicine that could cure old age?
   A. The medicine was too cheap. B. The medicine was too expensive.
   C. He looked quite old himself. D. He didn't look honest.
2. How much did the man charge for the cure for old age?
   A. One dollar a bottle. B. A hundred dollars a bottle.
   C. Ten dollars a bottle. D. Fifty dollars a bottle.

Structure

3. Another person cried, "Yes, you look ______ you are at least sixty years old."
   A. if B. as if C. as D. on
4. The man continued, "I'm not going to ______ you a hundred dollars a bottle ______ this wonderful medicine.
   A. spend... on B. cost... in C. charge... for D. spend... in
5. At first, he sold bottles of a cure ______ colds for just a dollar a bottle.
   A. for B. with C. by D. to
6. One person shouted, "If it will make you live forever, why ______ drink it? "
   A. will you B. won't you C. do you D. don't you

7. One of them spoke to the man's assistant ____ she passed by.

A. after B. before C. as D. for

Vocabulary

8. The crowd laughed at this.

A. was happy B. was sad C. made fun of D. was puzzled

9. "I'm going to charge you just ten dollars a bottle."

A. take B. cost C. spend D. expend

10. One of them spoke to the man's assistant as she passed by.

A. aide B. help C. companion D. associate

GRAMMAR FOCUS

1. —What should I do now? 我现在应该做什么呢?

—You should rub the ointment. 你应该擦这个药膏。

should 应该

e.g. You should consult your doctor. 你应该咨询你的医生。

2. — How often should I rub it? 我多久擦一次呢?

— When you needs. 当你需要的时候。

3. once a day 一天一次

twice a day 一天两次

three times a day 一天三次

4. after meals 饭后

before meals 饭前

with meals 随餐

empty stomach 空腹

at bedtime 睡前

Section B Extensive Reading

Ⅰ. Read the passage. Do you know "some medicine that can cure cancer"?

A New Cancer Drug

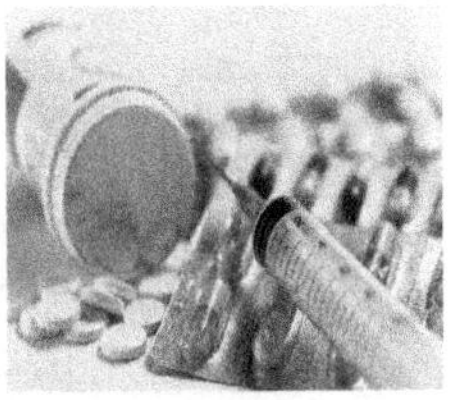

Scientists have developed a new cancer drug. So far, they have tested it only in laboratory animals. The drug is designed to enter and kill cancer cells, but not healthy cells.

First, the drug enters the cancer cells and stops their supply of blood.

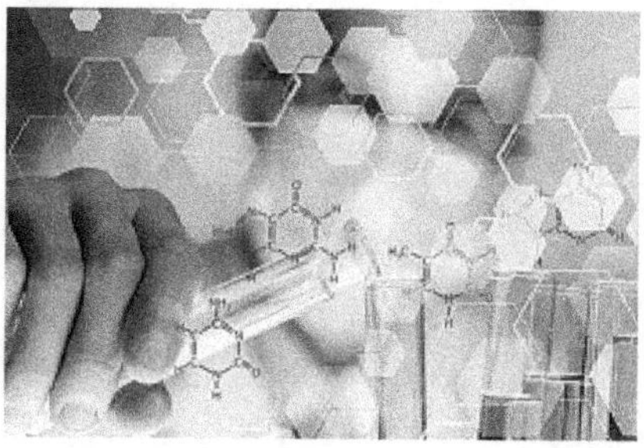

Then it releases poison to destroy the cancer cells.

Researchers in Cambridge carried out the study. A school report called the drug an "anticancer smart bomb". Ram Sasisekharan is one of those researchers. He says that his team had to solve three problems. They had to find a way to destroy the blood vessels, then to prevent the growth of new ones. But they also needed the blood vessels to supply chemicals to destroy the cancer.

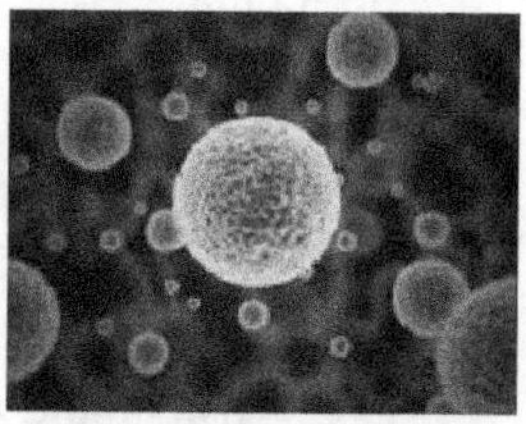

So, the researchers designed a two-part "nano-cell". The cell is measured in nanometer, or one thousand millionth of a meter.

The scientists said that it was small enough to pass through the blood vessels of the cancer, but it was too big to enter normal blood vessels. The surface of the nano-cells also helped them to avoid natural defenses.

The scientists designed the cell as a balloon inside a balloon. They filled the outer part with a drug that caused the blood vessels to die. That cut off the blood supply and put the nano-cells inside the cancer. Then, the nano-cells slowly released drugs to kill the cancer cells.

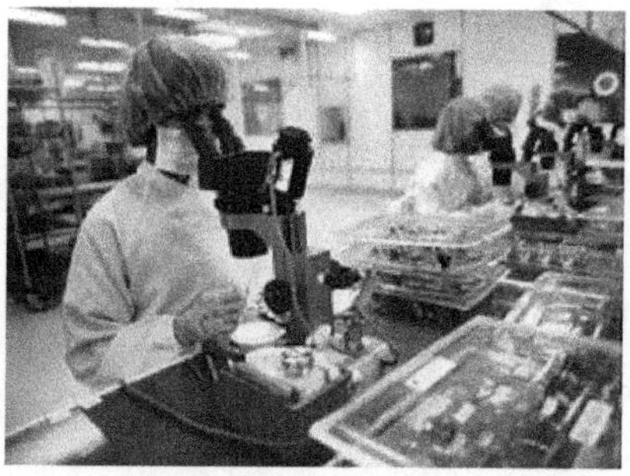

The team says that the treatment killed the cancer and avoided healthy cells better than other treatments. Untreated mice with cancer survived for twenty days. The scientists say that mice with the best current treatments lived for thirty days. In this study, they say that eighty percent of the mice treated with the nano-cells lived more than sixty-five days.

The scientists say that more studies are needed before the new drug can be tested on humans.

Ⅱ. Find out your unknown words and phrases in the text, written down and look up them.

Words	Meanings

Ⅲ. According to the passage, fill T for true or F for false.

1. ______ The drug is also designed to kill healthy cells.
2. ______ "nano-cell" is measured in millimeter.

3. ______ "nano-cell" can enter normal blood vessels.

4. ______ The mice treated with the nano-cells live longer than that mice treated with the best current treatments.

5. ______ The scientists say that the new drug can be used in humans.

Section C Writing

E-mail

电子邮件是一种电子化的信函，人们可以使用手机和电脑完成电子邮件的写、送、读。

SAMPLE

The following is an E-mail. Please read and try to understand it.

To: Allen_Green@gmail.com
Subject: Thanks!
From: Amy_Brown@yahoo.com
Date: July 21th, 2008

Dear doctor,

I am writing this letter to express my heartfelt thanks to you for your kind care and treatment when I was in hospital.

I remember when I was ill in bed; I was so worried about my condition. But your professional advice relieve my worries, the nurses on duty take care of me with great patience and tenderness, it is really kind of you all, now I have got a quick recovery. I feel great, thank you again for your professional service and kindness.

yours faithfully,
Amy

KNOWLEDGE

1．邮件头

邮件头包括发件时间（计算机完成）、收件人的e-mail地址（发件人输），寄件人的e-mail地址（计算机完成）和主题行（发件人输入）。主题行的内容应简明地概括信的内容，短的可以是一个单词，如greetings；长的可以是一个名词性短语，也可以是完整句，但长度一般不超过35个字母。主题行的内容切忌含糊不清。像News about the meeting这样的表达，应改为Tomorrow's meeting canceled。一般来说，只要将位于句首的单词和专有名词的首字母大写即可。

2．正文

e-mail文体的另外一个特点是简单明了，便于阅读，太长的内容可以以附件的方式发出。一个段落大多仅由一到三个句子组成。

3．签名

落款直接写发件人的姓名即可，如"yours Amy"。

EXERCISES

Fill in the blanks with the proper words.

To: Zhongshan_2005@yahoo.com
Subject: 1.______（预约）
From: Ella_2012@sina.com
Date: July 21, 2016
Dear Doctor Wang,

Thank you very much for your considerate service and 2.______（高超的技术）. I had an appendix 3.______（手术）5 days ago. Now I need to 4.______（换药）. May I make an appointment with you to change it? Please tell me when you are 5.______.（上班）

Thanks you once again, wish you success in your work, happy life!

yours faithfully,
Ella

Unit 6 Medical Examination

Section A *I Would Like to Make an Appointment to Have a Medical Examination on Friday.*

Language Goals: Talk about Making an Appointment to Have Body Check.

WARM-UP

Ⅰ. Match the phrases with pictures.

_______ CT

_______ blood pressure

_______ echoscope

_______ blood test

_______ B-mode ultrasonic exam

_______ pulse examination

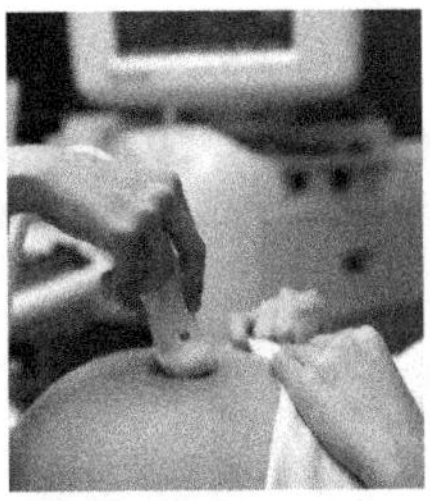
A

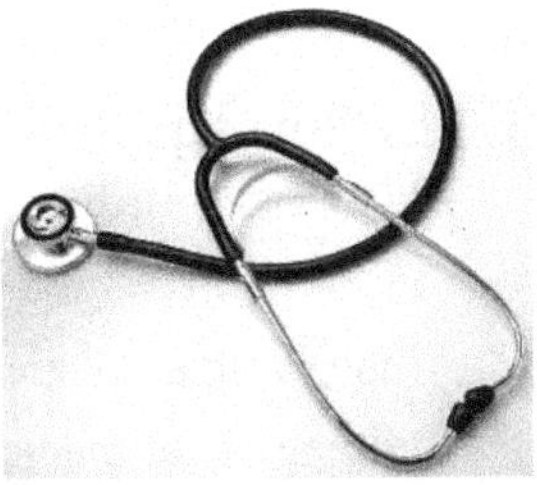
B

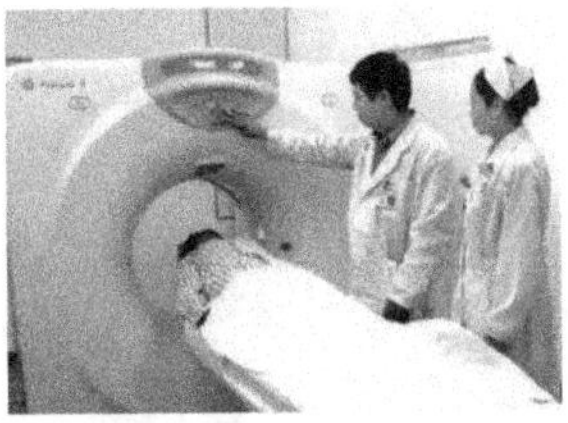
C

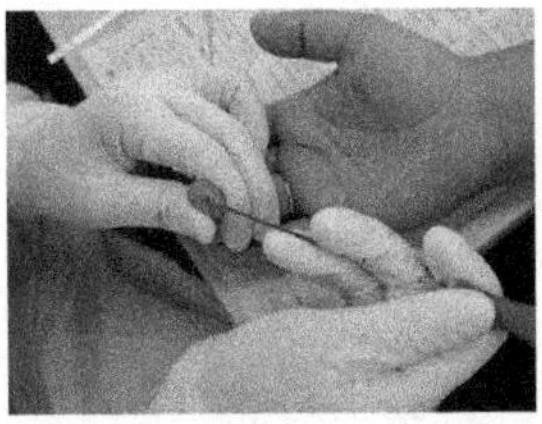
D

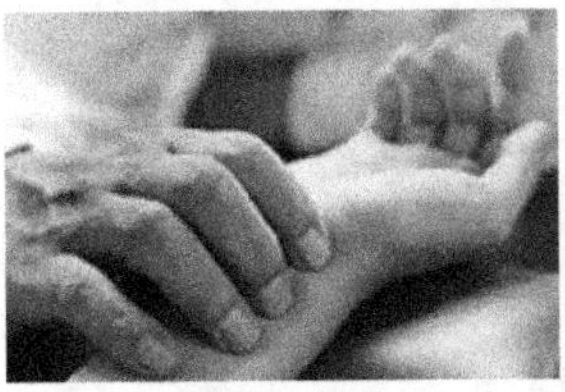
E

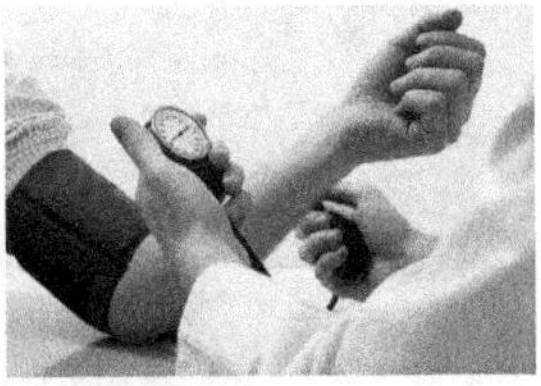
F

Ⅱ. Listen and number the pictures 1 to 4 in the order you hear them.

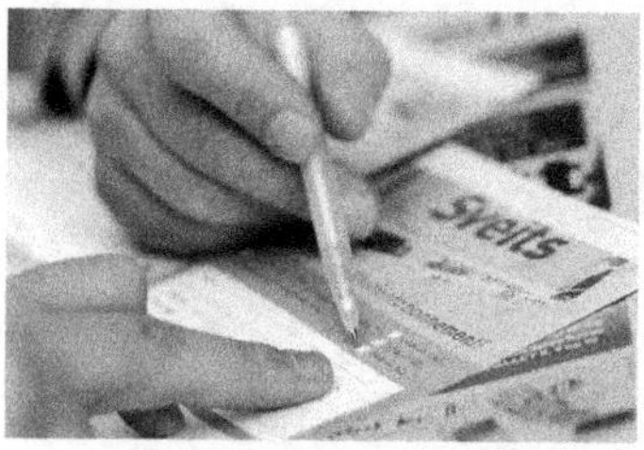

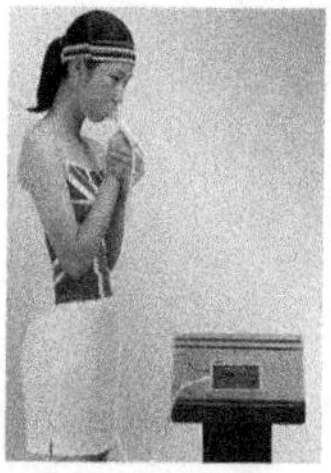

____ fill the health form

____ have lung capacity measurement

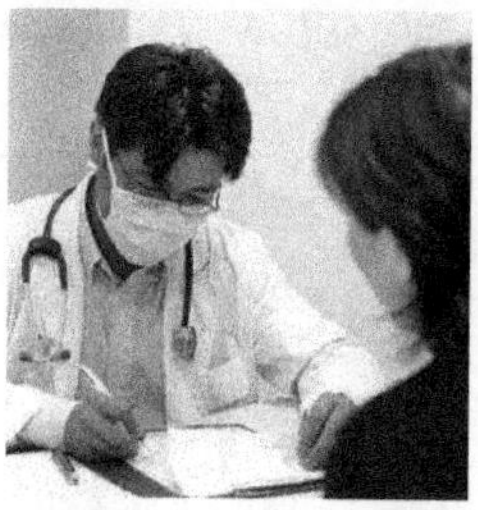

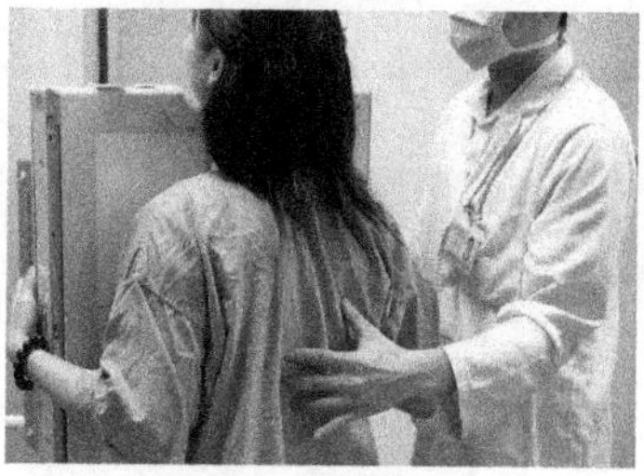

____ talk about medical history

____ take the chest X-ray

Ⅲ. Listen again and match the items with when they begin.

health form filling	begins at 7:00 am.
chest X-ray	begins at 8:30 am.
lung 's capacity measurement	begins at 9:00 am.
talking about medical history to doctors	begins at 11:00 am.

Ⅳ.Look at the pictures. Make conversations.

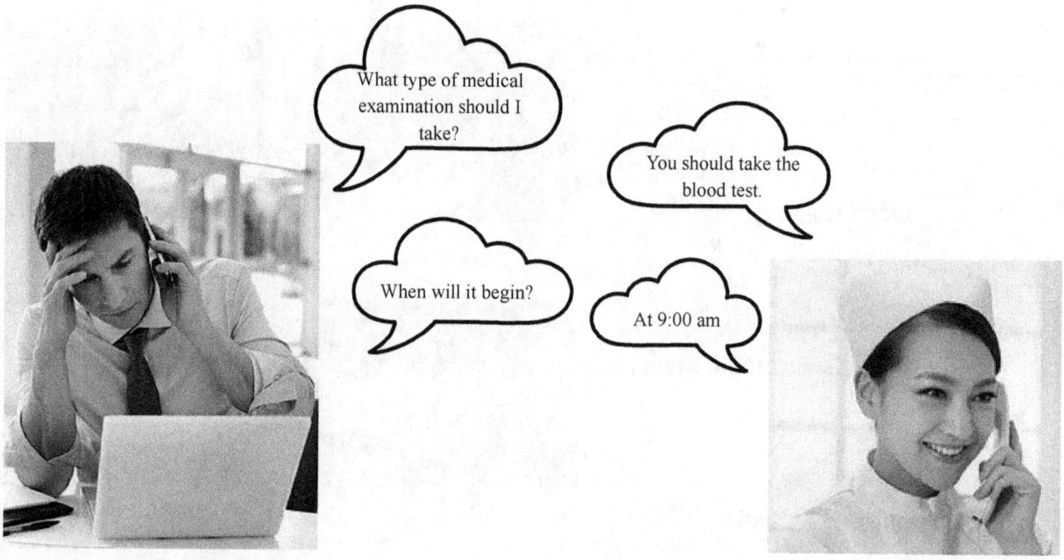
What type of medical examination should I take?
You should take the blood test.
When will it begin?
At 9:00 am

DIALOGUE

Role-play the conversation.

Nurse: Good afternoon.

Patient: Good afternoon, nurse. I would like to make an appointment to have a medical examination on Friday. Can you arrange it for me?

Nurse: Let me see. Friday is Ok. Please tell me your full name and phone number.

Patient: William Black. W-I-L-L-I-A-M, William, B-L-A-C-K, Black. My phone number is 13856977420.

Nurse: All right. Please be on time at 7:30.

Patient: How long will it take?

Nurse: The examination will last for about 3 hours. First, you should fill your health form on the first floor, and then you may go to take the blood test on the third flood. CT Room and Chest X-Ray Room are in the fourth floor. You can also find the guidelines in the lobby.

Patient: OK. Is there anything I should pay attention to?

Nurse: Oh yes. You had better not have breakfast before you have a blood test.

Patient: Thank you very much.

Nurse: You are welcome.

READING

Ⅰ. Read the passage and talk about why it is important for Medical Examination.

The Importance of Medical Examination

A medical examination is used to check your overall health. It examines many organs and other parts of your body, such as heart, lung, eyesight, stomach and so on.

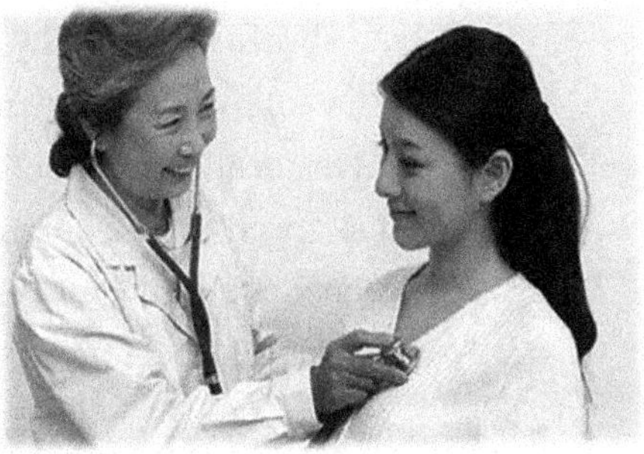

Annual physical examinations are important to prevent serious illness and ensure a long and healthy life for you and your family. Parents often make certain their children receive an annual examination; however exams become increasingly important into adulthood. There are typical exams you may experience at your annual exam, such as general appearance, heart exam, lung exam and so on.

To save your time, making an appointment is necessary before you go to have the examination. Both telephone appointment and online booking are wildly used in daily life. You should make a call or register on the Internet at least 24 hours prior to the coming time. You should give your personal information like your full name, gender, phone number and so on. What's more, you had better know clearly where to do each kind of examination.

During the examination, be honest to your doctor. Make sure you speak up with any questions or concerns you have about your health, no matter how minor they may seem. After examination, listen to your doctor's advice carefully and do not be shy to ask any questions.

There are two easy ways to prolong life for everyone: have annual medical examinations and live a healthy life. We should take measures to prevent illness whenever possible. Nothing can replace the importance of daily exercise, maintaining a healthy weight and not smoking.

Ⅱ. Find out your unknown words and phrases, written down and look up them.

Words	Meanings

Ⅲ. EXERCISES.

Reading Comprehension

1. The passage suggests that ______
   A. We don't need to see a doctor unless we have a serious illness.
   B. We can't make an appointment on the Internet.
   C. Medical examination is important.
   D. We can always keep healthy as long as we do exercise.
2. which of the following statements is true?
   A. Annual medical examination is very helpful for us to keep healthy.
   B. You don't need to give your personal information when making an appointment.
   C. You cannot tell the doctor you have drunk too much wine.
   D. You may not ask doctors any questions after examination.

Structure

3. Annual physical exams are important ______ preventing illness.

A. to B. for C. with D. on

4. You should make a call or register ______ the Internet.

A. to B. for C. with D. on

5. To save time, you can ______ an appointment before the exam.

A. make B. do C. play D. go

6. It is important for you to ______ honest to your doctor.

A. is B. be C. being D. are

7. You should do more exercise and have a balance diet if you want to ______ healthy.

A. feel B. make C. do D. keep

Vocabulary

8. Medical examination ______ many organs and other parts of the body.

A. examines B. examining C. see D. seeing

9. Annual physical exams are <u>important</u> for preventing illness.

A. big B. essential C. difficult D. different

10. <u>What's more</u>, you had better know clearly where to do each kind of exam.

A. However B. But C. And D. Moreover

11. Make sure you are honest to your questions or concerns and do not ______ .

A. tell a lie B. make a speech C. ask a question D. feel happy

GRAMMAR FOCUS

1. —I would like to make an appointment to have a medical examination on Friday. 我想预约星期五体检。

— Let me see. Friday is Ok. 让我看看。星期五可以。

类似的表达还有：How about /What about Thursday? 星期四可以吗?

Is Dr. Johnson available on Saturday? 约翰逊大夫周六有空吗?

2. — Please tell me your full name and phone number. 请告诉我你的全名和电话号码。

— William Black. W-I-L-L-I-A-M, William, B-L-A-C-K, Black. My phone number is 13856977420. 威廉·布莱克 . 我的电话号码是 13856977420.

类似的表达还有：Please tell me your own information. 请告诉我你的个人信息。

3. —How long will it take? 需要多长时间?

— The examination will lasts for about 3 hours. 体检将持续大概 3 个小时。

4. — Is there anything I should pay attention to? 我还需要注意什么吗?

Section B Extensive Reading

I. Read the passage. Do you know something about medical examinations in other countries?

Medical Examination Requirements for Visitors & Workers in Canada

If you plan to visit Canada for six months or less, a medical examination is not required. If you plan to visit for more than six months, you may have to get a body test. There are other situations where you also need to have this examination. For example, you have lived for six or more months continuously, or you will come to Canada to work in a job in which public health must be protected, or you want to apply for a Parent and Grandparent Super Visa.

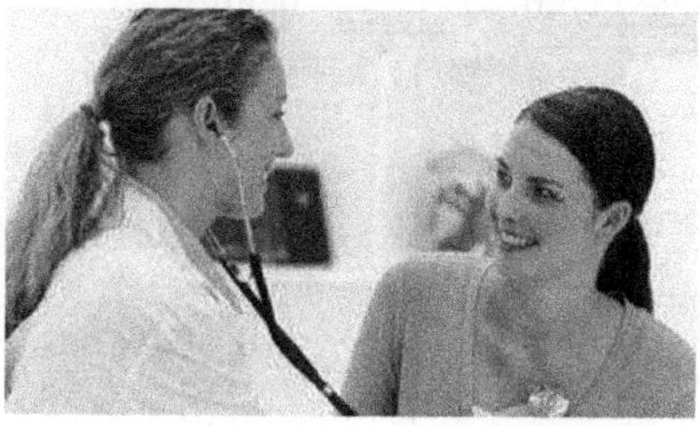

There are Jobs for which you need a medical exam:

1. Agricultural workers who have visited or lived in Canada for more than six months during the past year.

2. Jobs that bring you into close contact with people, such as:

a) workers in the health sciences field

b) clinical laboratory workers

c) teachers of primary or secondary schools, or other teachers of small children

d) workers who give in-home care to children, the elderly and the disabled

e) day nursery employees and other similar jobs

f) ...

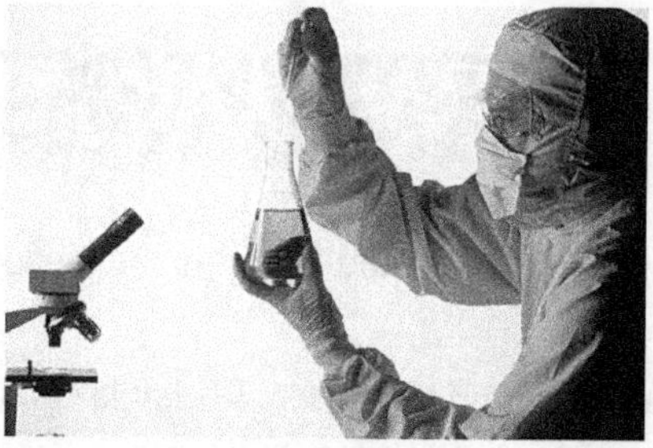

However, not all the doctors can perform the medical examination. You must see a doctor on the certain list of panel physicians. The panel physician will do a complete test to you. Once your examination is done, the physician will send you the results. If there is a problem with your health, the visa office will contact you in writing. If you want a copy of your medical examination result, please ask the doctor when you are there.

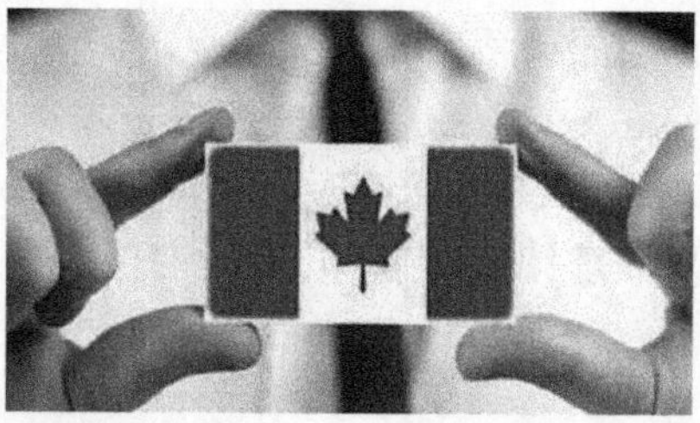

When it comes to fees, you must pay any fees related when you are there. If the government refuses your application after your medical examination, it will not refund those fees.

Ⅱ. Find out your unknown words and phrases in the text, written down and look up them.

Words	Meanings

Ⅲ. According to the passage, fill T for true or F for false.

1. ______ You do not need to have a medical examination if you plan to visit Canada for two months.
2. ______ Clinical laboratory workers should have medical examination in Canada.
3. ______ All the doctors can perform the medical examination.
4. ______ The panel physician will tell you the results after the examination.
5. ______ You can get fees back if the government refuses your application.

Ⅳ. Talk about your own experience about medical examination with your classmates.

Section C Writing

Memos

备忘录是一种用于公文备忘的文件。在公文函件中，备忘录的等级较低，主要用来提醒、督促对方或就某个问题提出自己的意见或看法。在业务上，它一般用来弥补正式文件的不足。它可以用便条书写，或者由公司制定统一格式的表格。

SAMPLE

The following is a memo of a hospital. Please read and try to understand it.

Memo

To: Ms. Johnson, Nurse superintendent of Inpatient Department
From: Lucy
Date: May 13th, 2017
Subject: Computer training course

In order to improve standard management and increase service quality of hospital, a course about nursing safety will be held from 3:00 pm to 6:00pm in May 20th, 2017 at the meeting room. Please be on time.

Cc: Alice

KNOWLEDGE

备忘录包括七个内容：

1. Heading：题目

在备忘录本文的上方正中央位置写下公文类型，即 Memo，也可写作 Memorandum。

2. Receiver：收笺人

收笺人前要加 To，并顶格。收笺人姓名前要加上 Mr. /Mrs. /Ms. 等，后面可加上收笺人的职位、部门。

3. Sender：发笺人

发笺人前要加 From，并顶格。需要注意的是，发笺人姓名前一般不加 Mr. Mrs. Ms. 等，后面也不加发笺人的职位、部门，如例文中直接写名字 Lucy 即可。

4. Date：日期

英文的日期通常以月、日、年为顺序，月份可以缩写，日和年之间用逗号隔开。

5. Subject: 主题

主题前面要加 Subject，并顶格。主题多采用不完整句子，只需少量几个词，甚至一个词表示，目的在于使收笺人对事项一目了然，便于及时处理。

6. Body: 正文

正文内容应简洁明了，若是活动通知，则要说明时间、地点、需要做的准备及其他注意事项。

7. Carbon copy recipients: 抄送人

抄送人前要加 Cc，并顶格。需要注意的是，和发笺人一样，姓名前一般不加 Mr. /Mrs./ Ms. 等，后面也不加发笺人的职位、部门，如例文中直接写名字 Alice 即可。

EXERCISES

Fill in the following form with the following information.

Memo

To: Mr. Smith

From: Ben

Date: August 9th, 2017

Subject: have a meeting about how to deal with doctor-patient relationship

1.______（由于）have a better understanding between doctors and patients, a meeting about 2.______（如何处理）doctor-patient relationship will be held 3.______（上午 9 点）in August 11 in 4.______（第四会议室）. Please be 5.______（准时）.

Unit 7 Admitted to Hospital

Section A *How Can I order a Hospital Bed?*

Language Goals: Talk about Inpatient Department, Making Reservation, Seeing a Doctor, and Describing Patient's Condition.

WARM-UP

Ⅰ. Match the phrases with pictures.

________ Doctor's office

________ Internal Medicine Departments

________ hospital bed

________ medical records

________ nursing notes

________ nurse station

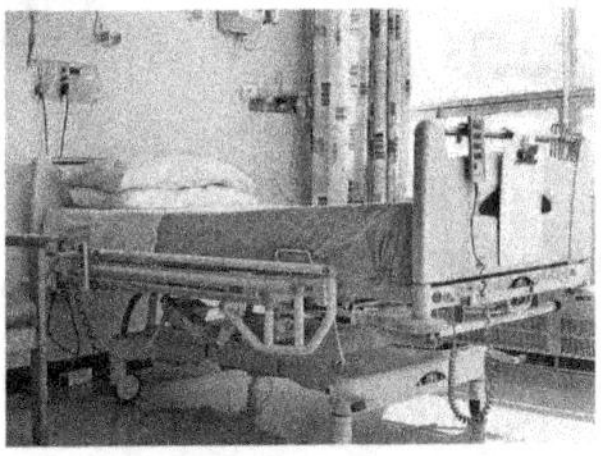

A

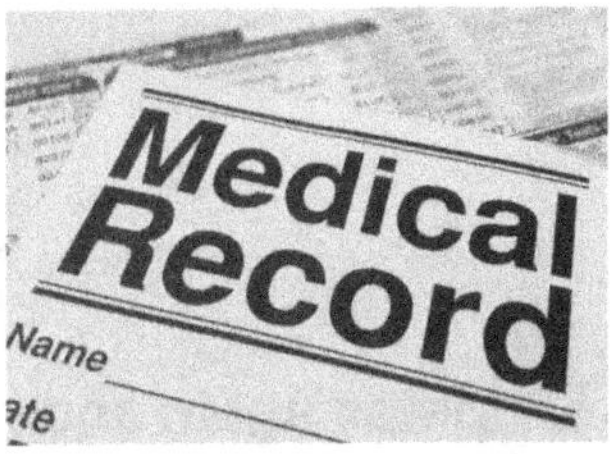

B

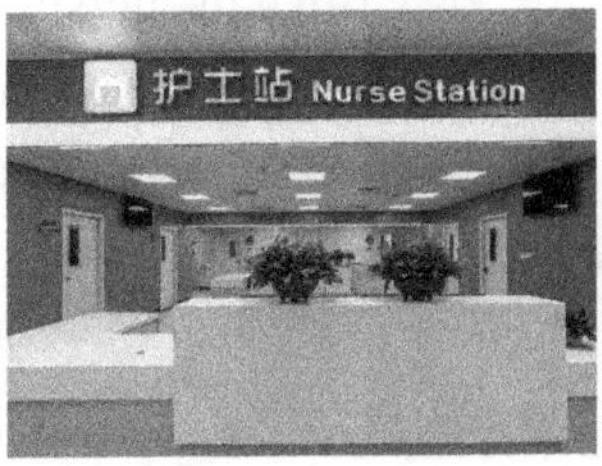

C

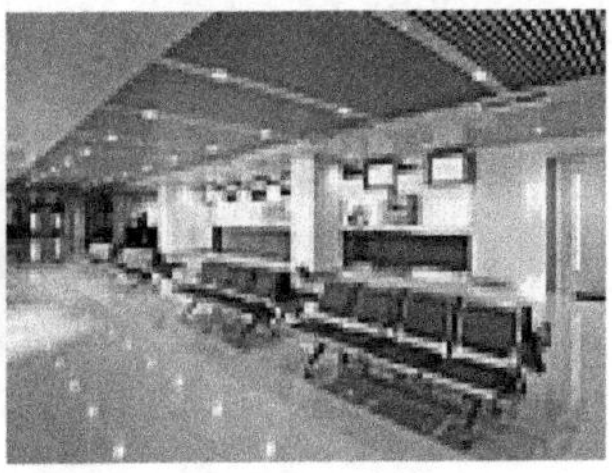

D

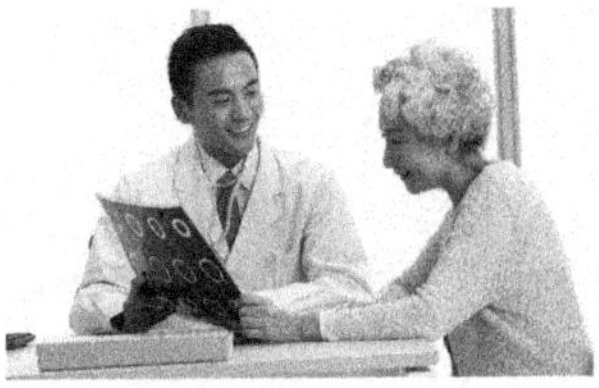

E

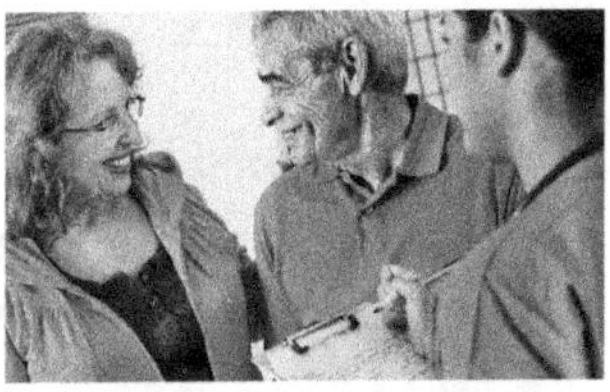

F

Ⅱ. Listen and number the pictures 1 to 4 in the order you hear them.

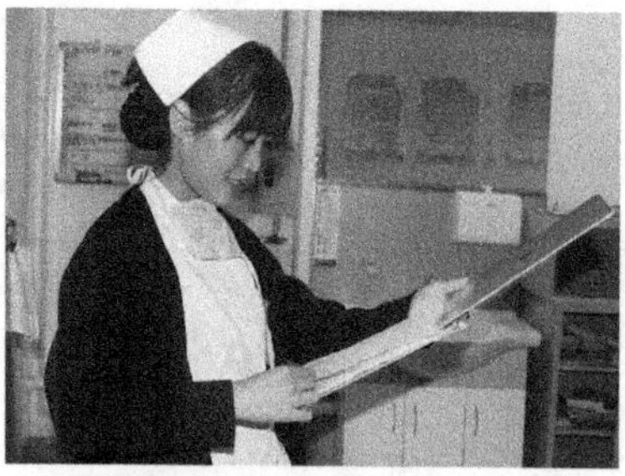

_____ checking the medical records

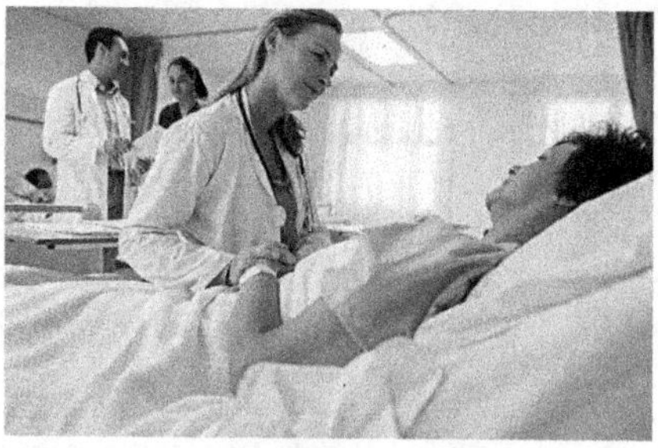

_____ reserving the hospital beds

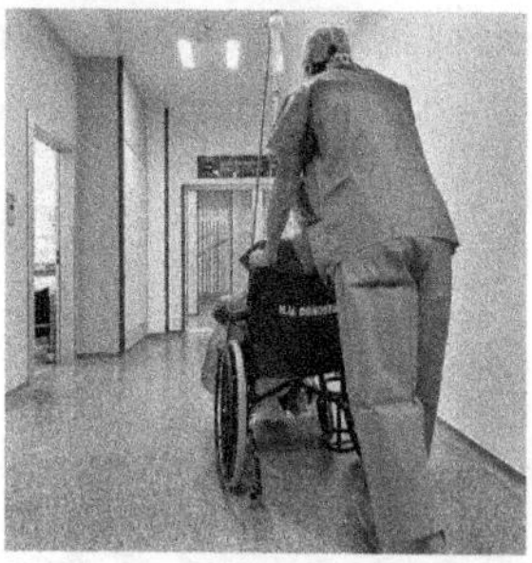

_____ transferring to the Internal Medicine Department

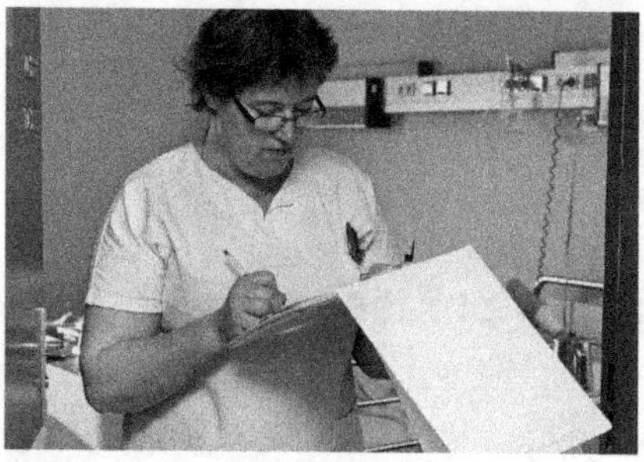

_____ writing the nursing notes

Ⅲ. Listen again and match the person with what they are doing now.

Lily	is transferring the patient to the Internal Medicine Department.
John	is writing the nursing notes.
Linda	is reserving the hospital beds.
Mary	is checking the medical records.

Ⅳ. Look at the pictures. Make conversations.

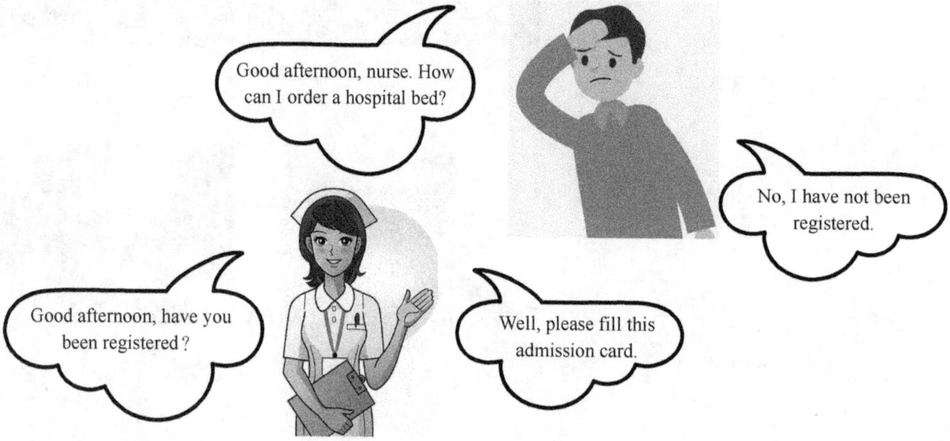
Good afternoon, nurse. How can I order a hospital bed?
Good afternoon, have you been registered?
No, I have not been registered.
Well, please fill this admission card.

DIALOGUE

Role-play the conversation.

Patient: Good morning, nurse. How can I order a hospital bed?

Nurse: Good morning, Sir. Have you been registered yet?

Patient: No, I have not been registered.

Nurse: Are you a medical or surgical case?

Patient: I'm a medical case.

Nurse: Do you have your history sheet?

Patient: Yes, here you are.

Nurse: Please, fill this admission card.

Patient: Oh, let me see... It is finished now.

Nurse: How long do you expect to stay in the hospital?

Patient: The doctor told me to stay about one month. I have nephritis. This is the second time to enter the hospital.

Nurse: Would you come to the hospital today?

Patient: Yes, I hope to enter the hospital this morning.

Nurse: But, there is no bed available now. This afternoon, two patients will be discharged. So you may be admitted this afternoon.

Patient: Well, when they leave the hospital, I shall admit.

READING

Ⅰ. Read the passage and tell "the admission procedure".

I was admitted into the hospital!

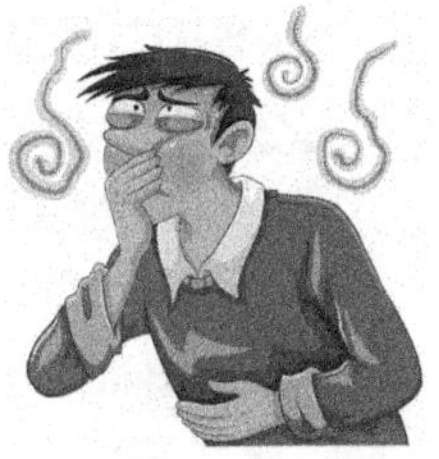

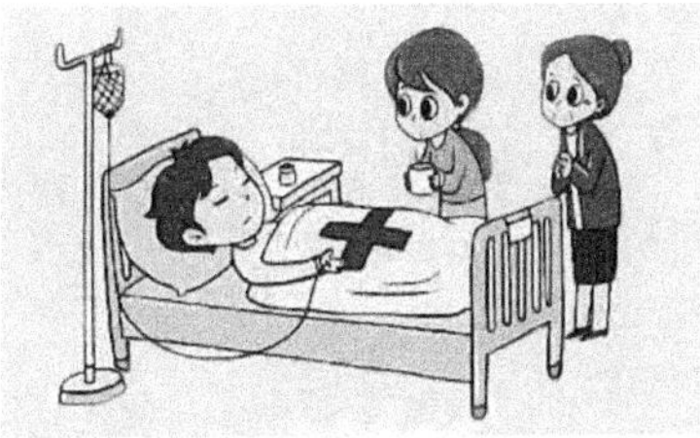

When I'm feeling ill or sick, I will go to the hospital to have a regular check-up in the outpatient department. Three days ago, I felt very sick and went to the hospital. After registration, I complained of having been vomiting for three days. The doctor gave me a physical examination and sent me to do some medical tests including blood tests, stool test and urine test. He told me that I was seriously ill and

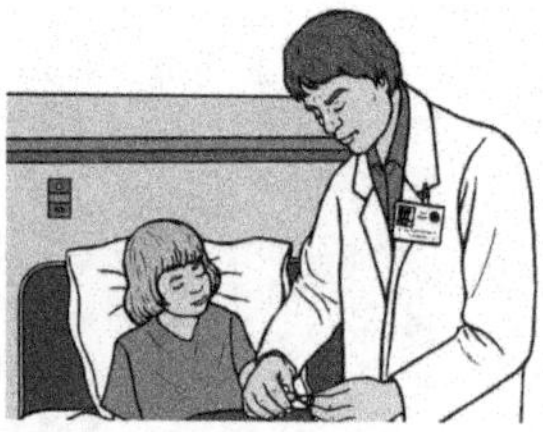

had to stay in hospital for further diagnosis or treatment. I followed the doctor's advice and got my admission notice from him.

I was asked to go through the admission procedure. Firstly, I showed my admission notice from my doctor to the nurse and then I went to the payment hall to pay the advance deposit.

After filling in the admission form and paying for the advance deposit, I was showed to my ward by a kind nurse. The nurse said to me, "Here is your ward; your bed number is 310A. This is the call light. Just push the button and a nurse will come to serve you immediately." She also reminded me that the visiting hours of the hospital are from 8:00 am to 8:30am, from 2:30pm to 3:00pm

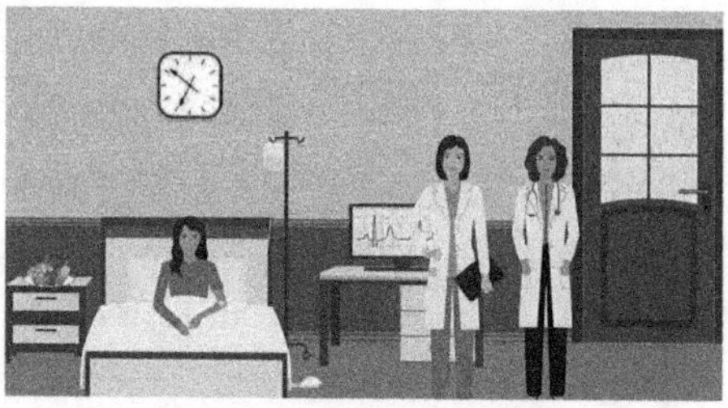

After a while, the ward nurse came to ask me if I am allergic to any medication, for example, penicillin. Actually, I have no idea. So the ward nurse did a skin test of penicillin for me. She also reminded me that if I felt itchy or short of breath, just let her know at once.

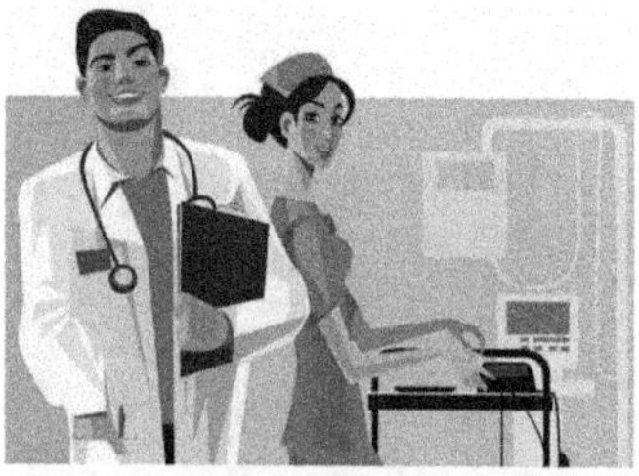

From the time I entered the hospital, my family and I had been looking forward to the day I was discharged. My symptoms and diseases were controlled because I actively cooperated with the treatment.

Ⅱ. Find out your unknown words and phrases, written down and look up them.

Words	Meanings

Ⅲ. EXERCISES.

Reading Comprehension

1.The story told us that ______ .

A.the author was ill and took some medicine at home.

B.the author filled in an application form.

C.the author paid the advance deposit for the family.

D.the author was seriously ill and was admitted into the hospital.

2. Which of the following statements is true?

A. I went into the hospital and complained of my headache.

B. I have got description from my doctor.

C. After filling in the admission form and paying for the advance deposit, I was showed to my ward by a kind nurse.

D. The doctor said he would carry me out an operation.

Structure

3. The doctor told me to stay ______ hospital for further diagnosis.

A. out B. in C. up D. to

4. — ______ did the author go to pay the advance deposit?

— The payment hall.

A. What B. How C. Where D. Why

5. After registration, the author complained ______ having been vomiting for three days.

A. of B. out C. to D. in

6. After admission into the hospital, the ward nurse came to ask me if I am allergic ______ any medication.

A. for B. to C. on D. from

7. The nurse reminded me ______ the visiting hours of the hospital are from 8:00 am to 8:30 am, from 14:30 pm to 15:00 pm.

A. to B. of C. that D. what

Vocabulary

8. When I'm feeling ill or sick, I will go to the hospital.

A. get an illness B. get angry C. feel unhappy D. feel comfortable

9. I will go to the hospital to have a regular check-up in the outpatient department.

A. skin test B. physical examination C. admission form D. nursing notes

10. I followed the doctor's advice and got my admission notice from the doctor.

A. followed the doctor's example B. followed the doctor's admission notice

C. took the doctor's advice D. wrote down the doctor's notes

11. The ward nurse did a ____ of penicillin for me.

A. skin test B. blood test C. medical report D. admission notice

GRAMMAR FOCUS

1. How can I order a hospital bed? 我怎样可以预定医院的床位?

order 作为动词，有订购、预定之意。order a hospital bed 预定床位；order breakfast 订早餐；He ordered three new suits for himself. 他给自己定购了三套西装。

2. — Have you been registered yet? 您挂号了吗?

— No, I have not been registered. 没有。我还没有挂号呢。

register 作为动词，表示登记、注册、挂号，名词形式为 registration。filling in the

registration form 填写登记表；What's your registration number? 你挂的是几号？

3. Are you a medical or surgical case? 您是挂内科还是外科？
   a medical case 内科病例、内科病人；a surgical case 外科病例、外科患者。
4. Do you have your history sheet? 您有病例单吗？
   history sheet 病历单。

e.g. All case history sheet paper has been used up. 病历表用纸都已经用完了。

5. There is no bed available, now. 目前没有床位了。
   available 作为形容词，表示可获得的、有空的。

e.g. This was the only room available. 只剩下那个房间可用了。

Section B Extensive Reading

Ⅰ. Read the passage. Have you ever heard "Admission to the Hospital"?

Admission to the Hospital

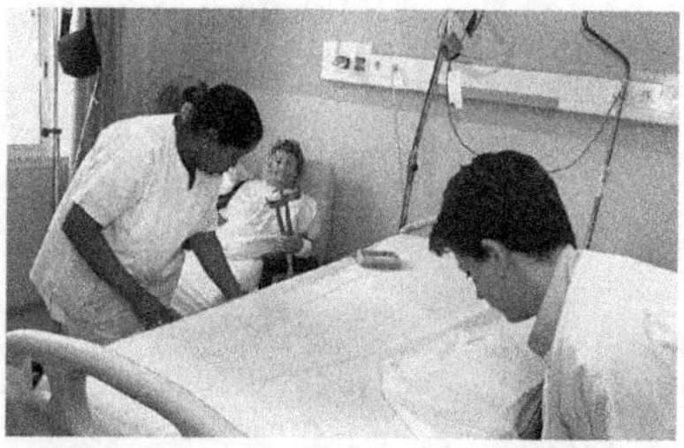

The admission of a patient is a formal process of entry into the hospital. To understand hospital procedures is very important when a patient is admitted to a hospital. The wards' environment, the nursing system will be introduced to the patients. What's more, inpatients' data will be collected to assess the clinical condition and nursing needs during the process.

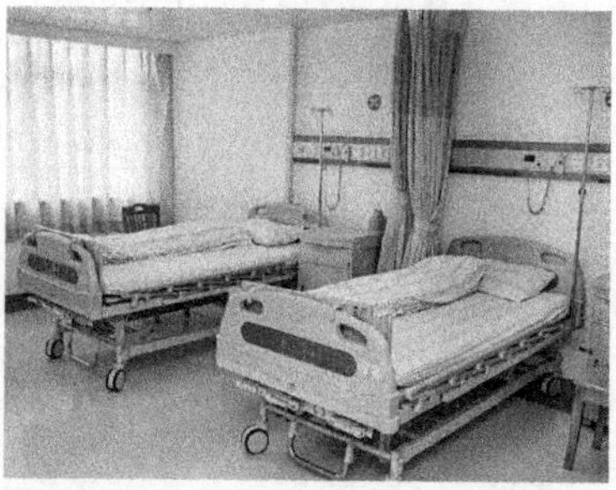

For the patients, admission card, admission form, ID card, National Health Insurance IC card and related certificates (major illness/injury card, etc.) as well as the previous medical records have to be checked when they are coming for admission. Admission card is given by the patient's attending doctor. The Admission form includes personal data, medical history, reason for admission, action to be taken, etc. The patient or his relative has to duly fill and sign the admission form prior to the admission. The medical history of a patient is information gained by a physician or other healthcare professionals by asking specific questions; either of the patient or of other people who know the person and can gives suitable information, with the aim of obtaining information useful in formulating a diagnosis and providing medical care to the patient.

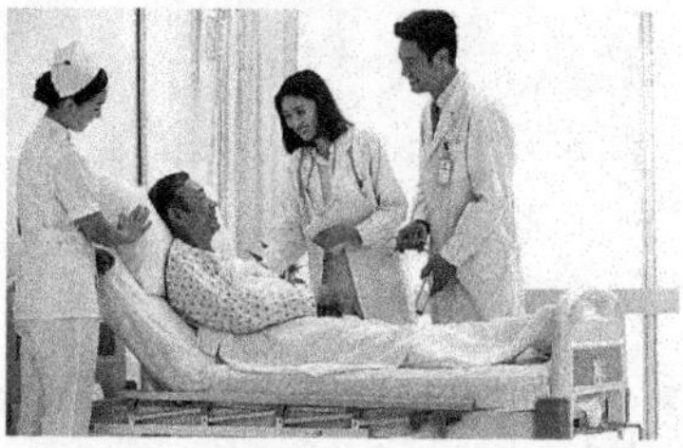

For the nurses, they should prepare the room when the admitting office tells the nurses that a patient is coming. The

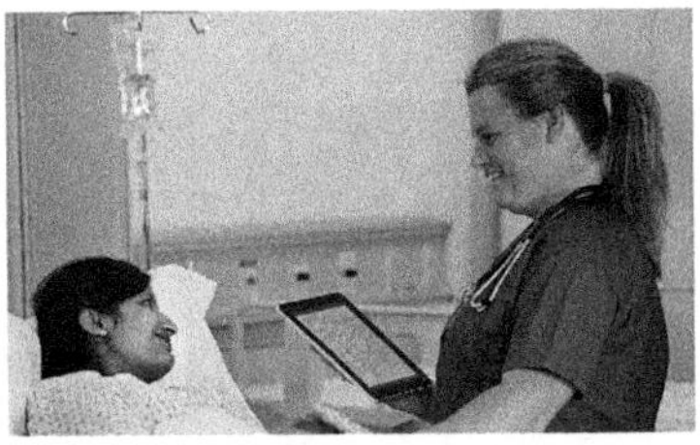

data of hospitalization will be informed by the nurses.

They settle inpatient procedures in the informed time or the beds would not be reserved.

The patient is never sent up to his room alone, because he might get lost or fall or be injured. As soon as the patient is admitted, the nurses should give him a physical examination. This is done because the hospital must have a complete record of the patient's condition.

Ⅱ. Find out your unknown words and phrases in the text, written down and look up them.

Words	Meanings

Ⅲ. According to the passage, fill T for true or F for false.

1. ______ To understand hospital procedures is very important when a patient is admitted to a hospital.

2. ______ Inpatients' data will be collected to assess the clinical condition and relatives' needs during the process of admission of a patient to the hospital.

3. ______ The admission form only includes medical history.

4. ______ The medical history of a patient is information gained by a physician or other healthcare professionals by asking specific questions.

5. ______ For the patients, they should prepare the room when the admitting office tells the patients that a nurse is coming.

Section C *Writing*

Diary Entries

日记是一种常见的私人写作形式，主要用于记录一天中的所见、所闻和所感。日记的形式简单，通常只需要在首行写明星期几、月 / 日 / 年和天气状况等基本信息即可。鉴于日记的私密性特点，其形式和内容在实际写作中具有很大的随意性。

SAMPLE

The following is a dairy entry. Please read and try to understand it.

September 22nd, 2017 Friday Sunny

The patient was called John Green, he was 16 years old. He was admitted into the hospital because of high fever, dry cough and no appetite on September 12th, 2017. Firstly, he was diagnosed as pneumonia and placed on erythromycin to dephlogisticate by attending physician Dr. William.

Until today, he has been in hospital for 10 days. His condition has improved a lot. The patient had good appetite this morning and showed general state of health. Based on his recent condition, he will be discharged the day after tomorrow according to the doctor's advice.

At last, he was diagnosed as pneumonia and Dr. William told the patient that no medications needed after discharge.

KNOWLEDGE

1. 日期表达有多种形式

年、月、日都写时，通常以月、日、年为顺序，月份可以缩写，日和年之间用逗号隔开。例如：December 18th, 2003 或者 Dec.18th, 2003。

2. 星期的表达

星期也可以省略不写，可将其放在日期前或后，星期和日期之间不用标点，但要空一格，星期也可缩写。如：Saturday, October 22nd, 2004；October 22nd, 2004 Saturday。

3. 天气情况必不可少

天气一般用一个形容词表示，如 sunny, fine, rainy, snowy 等。天气写在日期之后，用逗号隔开，位于日记的右上角。

4. 时态

日记中所记述的事情通常发生在过去，常用一般过去时；但当记述天气、描写景色或展望未来时，可以用一般现在时或一般将来时。

EXERCISES

Supposing today is Monday. The date is October 16, 2017. It is a rainy day. You are the ward nurse Wang Ling. Please write a diary about your day taking care of the inpatient Michael Smith according to following information:

Date: ______ Weather: ______

The patient was called 1. ________（米歇尔·史密斯）, he was 18 years old. He was 2. ________（入住到）the hospital because of 3. ________（呕吐）on 4. ________（2017 年 10 月 16 日）. His attending physician was Liu Tao. He was diagnosed as acute gastroenteritis. The patient was admitted and placed on fluid rehydration and mineral supplement.

Until today, he has been 5. ________（住院）for 5 days. The patient 6. ________（改善，好转）, showing gradual resolution of 7. ________（恶心 / 作呕 / 反胃）and vomiting.

Based on his recent condition, he will be discharged tomorrow 8. ________（遵医嘱）. The doctor told the patient that no 9. ________（药物 / 用药）will be needed 10. ________（出院后）. But if this patient can not get used to Chinese food, he had better return to USA as soon as possible to prevent the relapse of acute gastroenteritis.

Unit 8

Discharging from the Hospital

Section A My Discharge Summary is No See.

Language Goals: Talk about Discharging from the Hospital. Ask for Help.

WARM-UP

Ⅰ. Match the phrases with pictures.

________ discharge summary

________ diagnosis

________ doctor in charge

________ ward-round

________ disinfection

________ bed-making

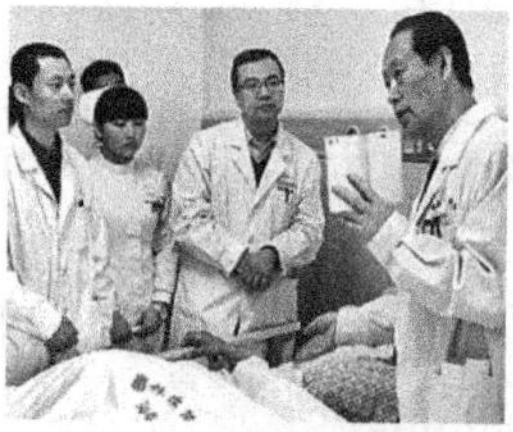
A

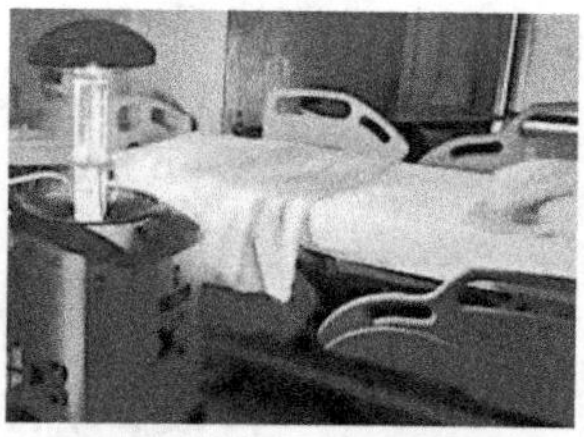
B

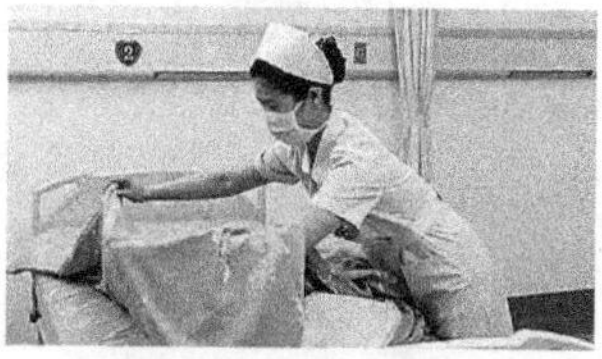
C

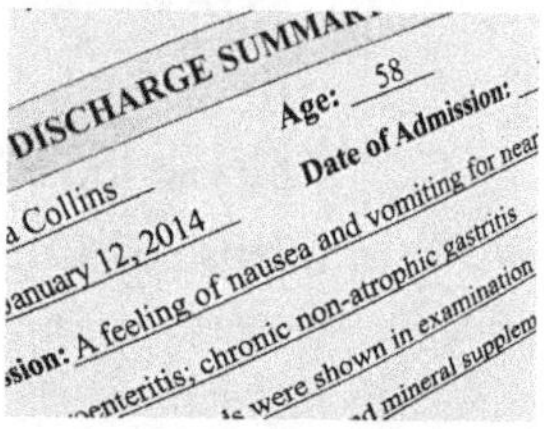

D

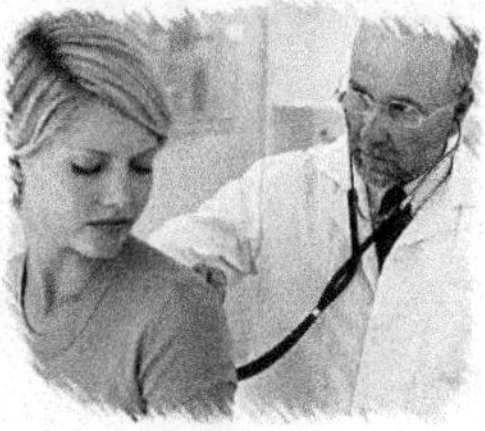
E

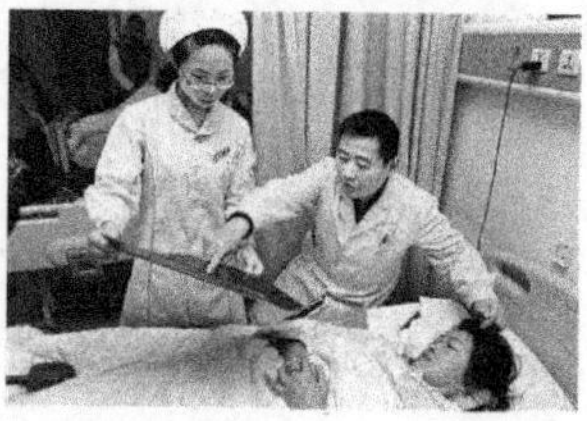
F

Ⅱ. Listen and number the pictures 1 to 4 in the order you hear them.

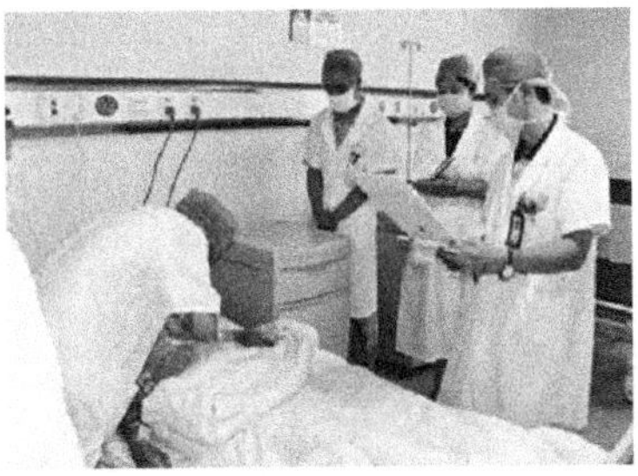

______ make a ward-round

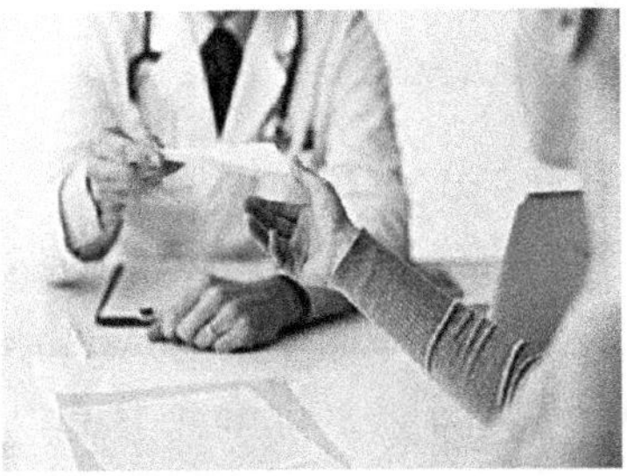

______ give a medication instruction

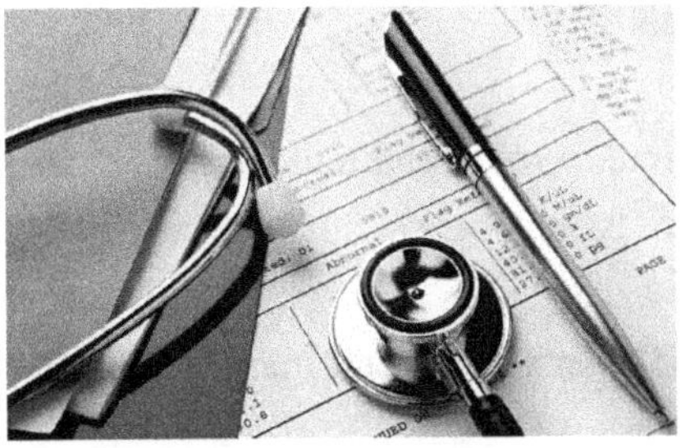

______ complete the discharge summary

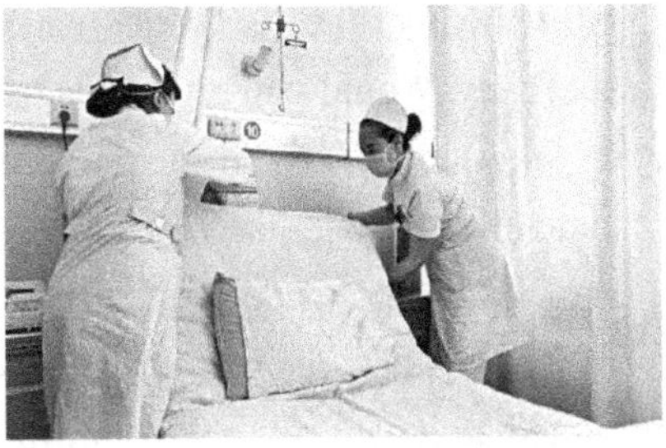

______ tidy up the ward

Ⅲ. Listen again and match the nursing intervention with time.

makes a ward-round	before the patients leave the hospital
gives medication instructions	after the patients leave the hospital
completes discharge summaries	from 9:00 am to 10:00 am
tidy up the wards	after the ward-round

Ⅳ. Make conversations.

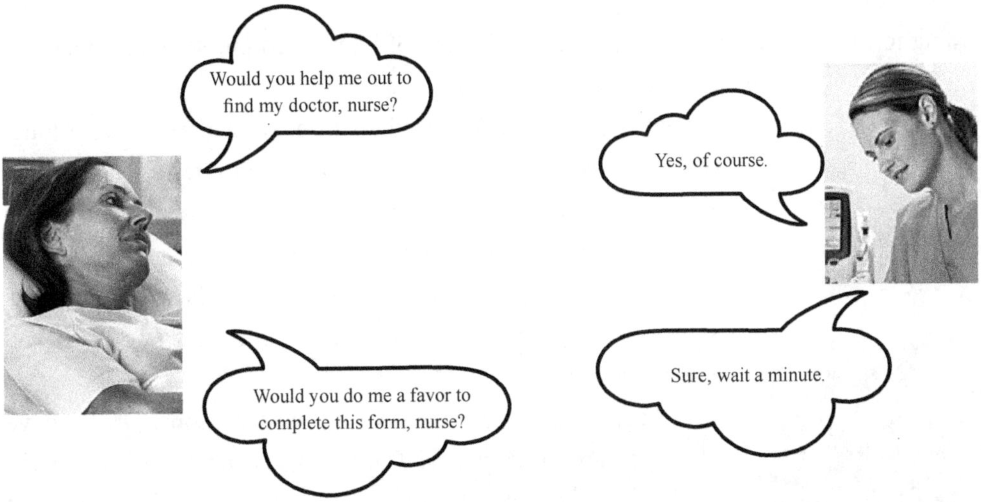
Would you help me out to find my doctor, nurse?
Yes, of course.
Would you do me a favor to complete this form, nurse?
Sure, wait a minute.

DIALOGUE

Role-play the conversation.

Patient: Good morning, doctor. Would you help me, please?

Doctor: Sure, Mr. Li. what's wrong with you?

Patient: My discharge summary is no see. I'm worried about my discharging from the hospital.

Doctor: Don't worry, I will see to it. This is your new discharge summary. Here you are. Do you still remember the discharge instructions?

Patient: Not really. Would you give me a hand?

Doctor: My pleasure. Take the medicine on time. Avoid drinking alcohol. Leave bed and do some exercise with the help of your family members at home, if possible.

Patient: Ok, I'll try. And what else?

Doctor: Try to do whatever you can but never push yourself too hard. Return to the hospital immediately whenever uncomfortable.

Patient: OK. Thank you for everything you've done for me, doctor.

READING

Ⅰ. Read the passage and discuss about "Mr. Li's Hospitalization".

Mr. Li's Hospitalization

A week ago, Mr. Li was admitted in the hospital because of the serious dizziness, blurred vision and chest pain.

According to Mr. Li's complaint, he had a long history of high blood pressure. His doctor in charge, Dr. Lu, decided to give him a complete examination.

In the first three days, Mr. Li was busy with different kinds of examinations. Before long, all necessary examinations were completed after the admission. Results of examinations such as blood routine, fecal routine, urine routine, coagulation routine, chest X-ray and ECG were normal. Color Doppler ultrasound was used in those examinations as well. And the results of it indicated Mr. Li's fatty liver and arteriosclerosis.

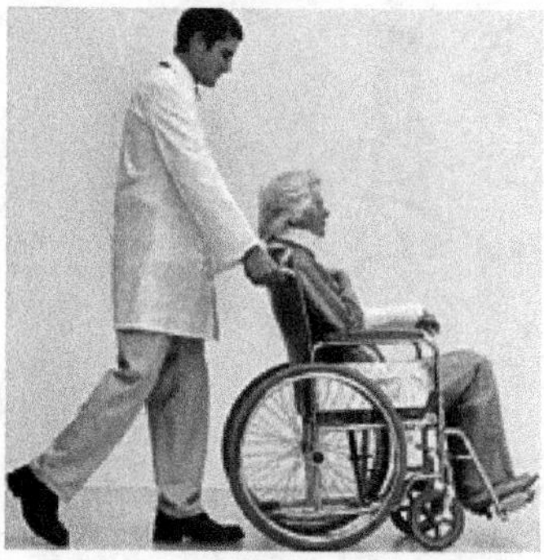

According to the results of all examinations, Dr. Lu gave Mr. Li a careful diagnosis. The necessary measures were taken for Mr. Li during the hospitalization. Measures for improving circulation, controlling blood pressure and improving mood and sleep were taken to Dr. Lu's instructions. And that really worked for relieving Mr. Li's pain and pressure.

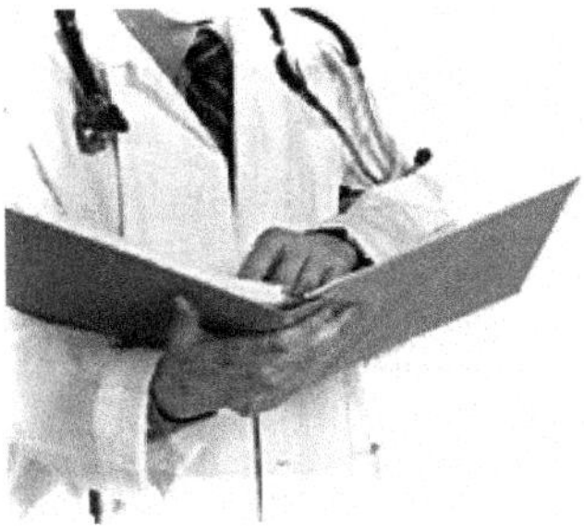

With the careful treatments and nursing, Mr. Li's mood and sleep was improved. His dizziness, blurred vision and chest pain were relieved. His general status was much better and he became more and more optimistic.

Ⅱ. Find out your unknown words and phrases, written down and look up them.

Words	Meanings

Ⅲ. EXERCISES.

Reading Comprehension

1. What necessary examinations were NOT completed after Mr. Li's admission? ______
   A. blood routine B. fecal routine
   C. chest X-ray D. thyroid function
2. Which statements are NOT true? ______
   A. The result of chest X-ray is normal.
   B. The result of coagulation routine is normal.
   C. The results of Color Doppler ultrasound are normal.
   D. The result of ECG is normal.

Structure

3. A week ago, Mr. Li was admitted in the hospital because ______ serious dizziness, blurred vision and chest pain.
   A. in B. on C. that D. of
4. According ______ Mr. Li's complaint, he had a long history ______ high blood pressure.
   A. to, in B. to, of C. in, of D. in, to
5. In the first three days, Mr. Li was busy ______ different kinds ______ examinations.
   A. with, in B. to, with C. with, of D. in, to
6. ______, all necessary examinations were completed after the admission.

A. Long before B. Long long ago

C. Long ago D. Before long

7. Color Doppler ultrasound was used in those examinations ______ .

A. as far B. as good C. as well D. as much

Vocabulary

8. And the results of it ______ Mr. Li's fatty liver and arteriosclerosis.

A. shown B. suggesting C. indicated D. mentions

9. The necessary measures were taken for Mr. Li during the ______ .

A. hospital B. hospitalization C. hospitalize D. hospitalized

10. And that really ______ relieving Mr. Li's pain and pressure.

A. worked for B. worked to C. worked in D. worked out

GRAMMAR FOCUS

1. Would you help me? Would you give me a hand? Would you help me out to... ? Would you do me a favor to...?

上述四个句型都可用于表示"你能帮帮忙吗？"

2. My discharge summary is no see. 我的出院小结不见了。

3. Don't worry, I will see to it. 别担心，我来处理。

see to...，处理、照料。

4. Do you still remember the discharge instructions? 还记得出院医嘱的内容吗？

5. Not really. Would you give me a hand? 记不太清楚了。你能帮帮忙吗？

6. My pleasure. Take the medicine on time. Avoid drinking alcohol. Leave bed and do some exercise with the help of your family members at home, if possible. 很荣幸。请按时吃药。避免饮酒。如果可以，在家人的帮助下离床做做运动。

7. Try to do whatever you can but never push yourself too hard. Return to the hospital immediately whenever uncomfortable. 能做到的事尽量去做，但不要太勉强。如有任何不适，立即回院就诊。

Section B Extensive Reading

I. Read the passage. Learn about Discharge Instructions.

Discharge Instructions					
Name	Li Yuan	Age	68	Gender	Male
Department	Neurology	Bed No.	5	Admission Number	1407151
Date of Discharge	June 20th, 2014	Status on Discharge		No headache or short-breath. Spirit, appetite and sleep is well. Normal urine and stool.	

Continued

Dos and Don'ts
1. Take enough rest and adequate exercises.
2. Avoid getting fatigued and catching cold.
3. Monitor carefully the intake of sodium and lipids in diets. 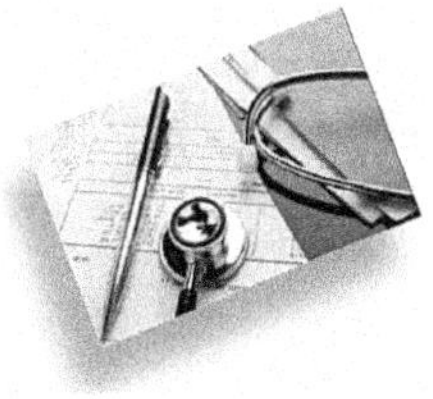
Discharge Medications
1. Benazepril tablets (10mg, po, qd);
2. Pregabalin capsules (75mg, po, qn);
3. Alprazolam tablets (0.4mg, po, qn). 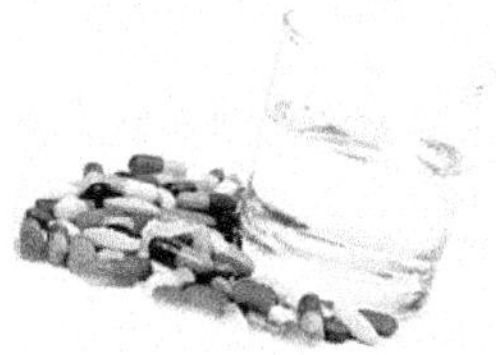
Instructions
1. Monitor blood pressure and blood lipids.
2. Use Color Doppler ultrasound to take the routine examinations of liver and artery.
3. Return to the hospital for examinations regularly and whenever uncomfortable.
Doctor's Signature: Lu Di

Ⅱ. Find out your unknown words and phrases in the text, written down and look up them.

Words	Meanings

Ⅲ. According to the passage, fill T for true or F for false.

1. _______ Take less rest and more exercises.
2. _______ Monitor the intake of sodium and lipids in diets randomly.
3. _______ Alprazolam tablets (10mg, po, qd).
4. _______ Monitor blood pressure and heart rates.
5. _______ Take routine examinations of liver and artery.

Ⅳ. Recite the doctor's instructions, rewrite it into a short conversation and role play it.

Section C *Writing*

Nursing Notes

Nursing Notes (护理记录) 用于反映患者生病住院期间的全部医疗护理情况，是临床教学和科研工作中不可缺少的重要资料。此类医疗文件具有很强的法律效力。

SAMPLE

The following is a part of nursing notes. Please read and try to understand it.

Nursing Notes					
Name	Hu Han	Age	65	Gender	Female
Department	Surgery	Bed No.	2	Admission Number	1703151
Date & Time			9:00 May 20th, 2014	9:00 May 21st, 2014	
Vital signs	Temperature	℃	38	36	
	Pulse	Time/min	65	60	
	Respiratory	Time/min	20	19	
	Blood Pressure	mmHg	120/64	115/70	
SpO_2		%	97	100	
Catheter and drainage tube			✓	✓	
Intake	Volume ml		250	400	
Output	Volume ml		100	300	
Others			N	N	
Signature			Li Yang	Mu Yan	
Explanation: If nothing has been observed, sign the blank with "N".					

KNOWLEDGE

护理记录是护理病历的核心部分，集护理计划、护理措施、措施依据、效果评价为一体。针对不同患者的不同病症，护理记录应翔实、具体地记录以下内容：

1．医疗数据及信息

此类消息包括所采取的治疗措施和护理措施，措施采取后的效果及不良反应；实验室检查的阳性结果、护理措施操作时间、关键步骤、临时给药的药品名称和剂量、患者的反应等。

2．生命体征、医嘱执行情况及一般患者的出院指导

重点记录生命体征及医嘱观察的内容。在一般患者出院前，写明病情、转归情况以及需要向患者及家属交代的健康问题。

3．手术患者的护理记录及出院指导

对于手术患者，应记录患者术前准备及病情变化等情况；术后前 3 天随时记录病情变化。出院当天记录患者术后伤口情况，有无引流管、拆线。需要向患者及家属交代院外饮食、休息、用药、复查及相关的预防保健知识和注意事项。

EXERCISE

Fill in the following form with the given information.

外科住院部 13 床病人李越，住院号 1703051，男，45 岁。2017 年 7 月 18 日上午 10:00 查房，生命体征平稳：体温 36.2 摄氏度，脉搏 76 次 / 分，呼吸 18 次 / 分，血压值 120/80。血氧饱和度 99。有导流管，入量 800 毫升，出量 200 毫升。无其他情况。护士刘芳签名记录。

Nursing Notes				
Name	Li Yue	Age	Gender	
Department		Bed No.	Admission Number	
Date & Time				10:00 July 19th, 2017
Vital signs	Temperature	℃		36
	Pulse	Time/min		60
	Respiratory	Time/min		19
	Blood Pressure	mmHg		115/70
SpO_2		%		100
Catheter and drainage tube				✓
Intake	Volume ml			400
Output	Volume ml			300
Others			N	N
Signature			Liu Fang	Yu Yan

Explanation: If nothing has been observed, sign the blank with “N” .

Unit 9

Health Education

Section A You Should Eat Fluids.

Language Goals: Talk about the Health Care and Health Guidance for Diseases.

WARM-UP

I. Match the things with pictures.

________ fluids

________ traction

________ massage

________ supine position

________ lung capacity

________ balance exercises

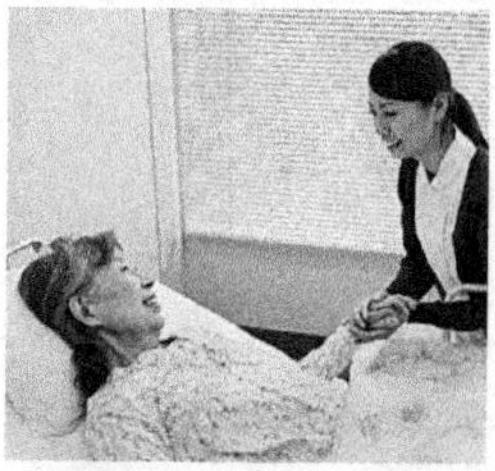

A

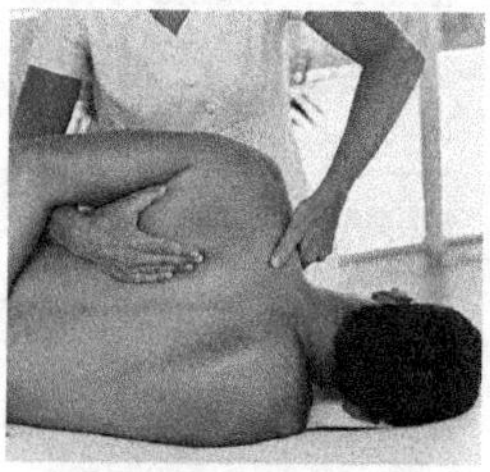

B

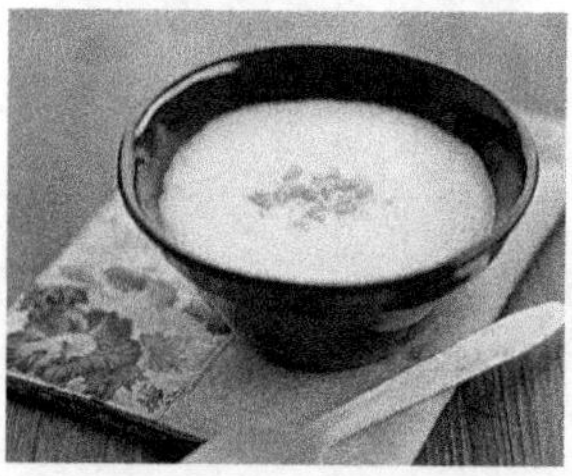

C

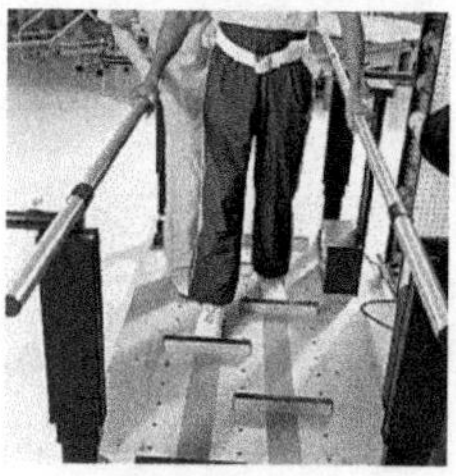

D

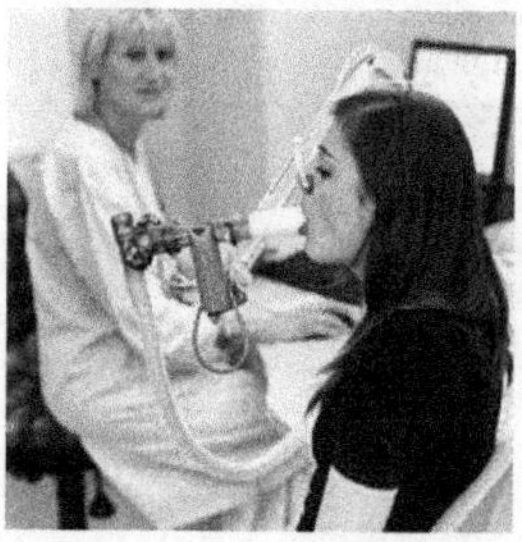

E

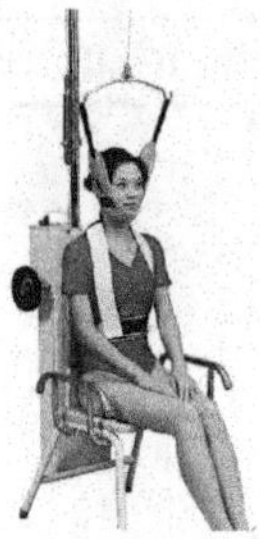

F

Ⅱ. Listen and number the pictures 1 to 4 in the order you hear them.

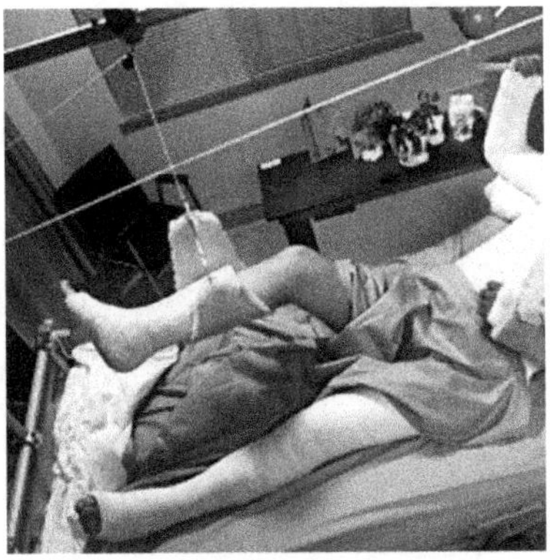

_______ be in traction

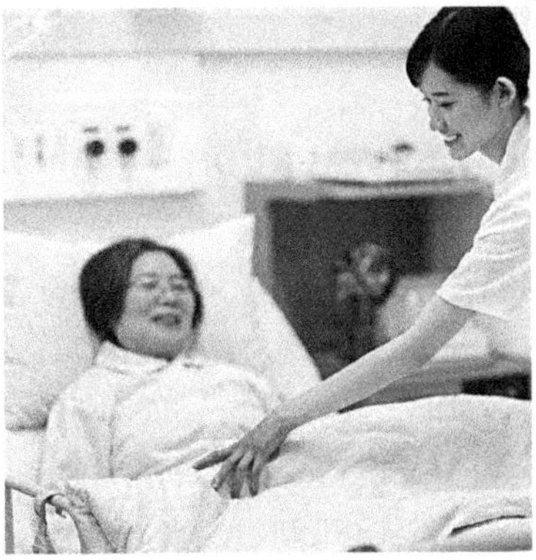

_______ sleep in supine position

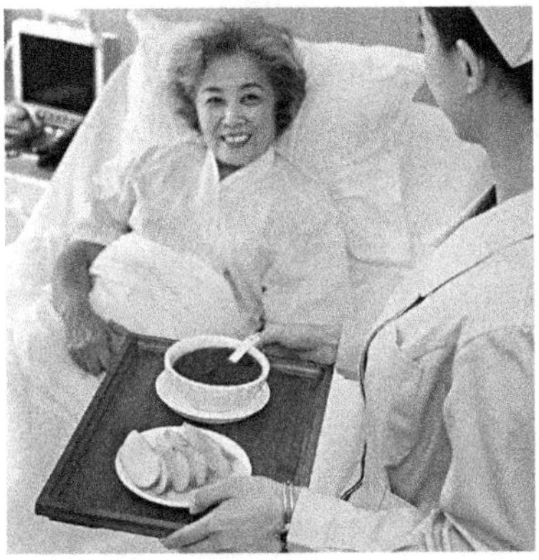

_______ eat fluids

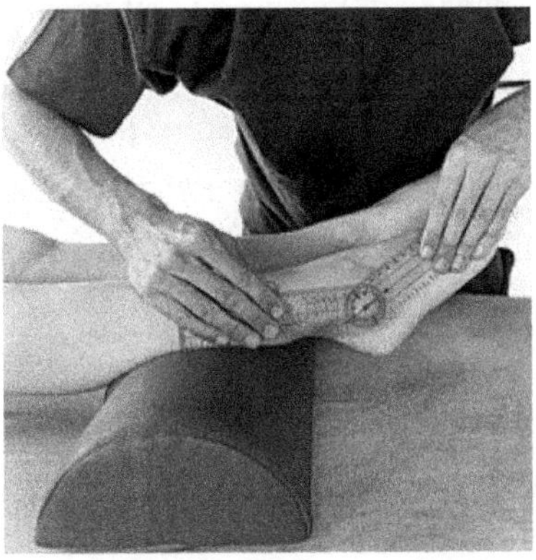

_______ go for a massage

Ⅲ. Listen again and match the therapy method with health guidance.

sleep in supine position	to help the recovery
eat fluids	to promote the blood circulation
be in traction	to avoid choke
go for a massage	to be easy for absorption

Ⅳ. Look at the pictures. Make conversations.

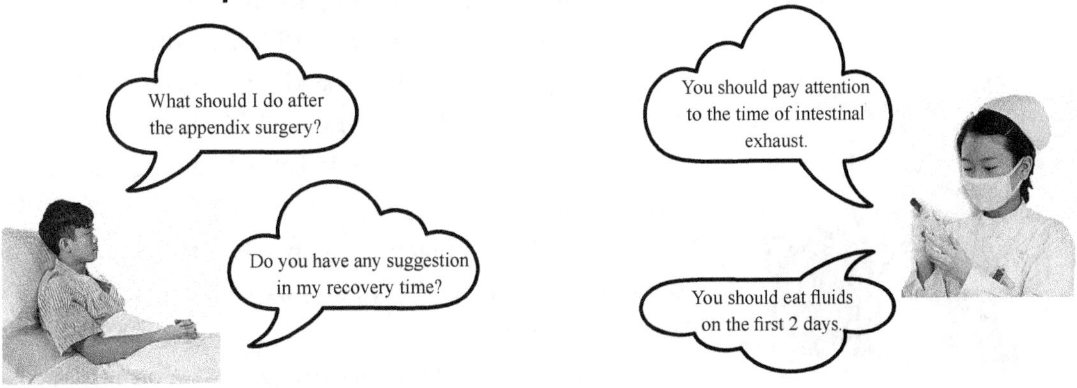
What should I do after the appendix surgery?
Do you have any suggestion in my recovery time?
You should pay attention to the time of intestinal exhaust.
You should eat fluids on the first 2 days.

DIALOGUE

Role-play the conversation.

Nurse: Good morning, Frank. You must know you'll have an operation next morning.

Patient: Good morning, nurse. Yes, I knew. What should I do before the operation?

Nurse: You should be NPO after 10 O'clock tonight, because your operation will start at 9 O'clock tomorrow morning.

Patient: Ok. What about my diet today?

Nurse: You should eat fluids today, Frank.

Patient: Yes, I'll follow your advice. And is there anything I should pay attention to?

Nurse: You need to tell us if you feel uncomfortable before the operation.

Patient: Yes, I will. Do you have any advice for me after the operation?

Nurse: You'd better sleep in supine position in the first 6 hours after operation. And you should be up and about in the first 24 hours.

Patient: I will. I have learned a lot from your advice, thank you so much, nurse!

Nurse: It's my duty. Goodbye, Frank.

READING

Ⅰ. Read the passage and tell "How to stay healthy".

It's Too Early to Lose Weight

Bill is a painter. He is an overweight man. He is always being stressed for his job.

One day, Bill felt uncomfortable and came to the hospital. Doctor diagnosed Bill and found he would be ill for his overweight.

"You should try to lose weight, sir." Doctor advised him, "Obesity is an important cause of high blood pressure. And high blood pressure may be harmful to your health."

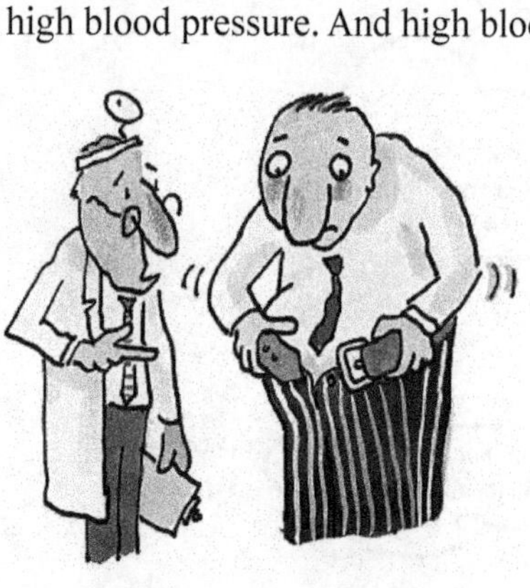

"What should I do, doctor? " Bill said sadly.

"Remember, the chair is the killer." Doctor said to Bill, "Do not sit for a long time. You should take more exercise and should not stay up late, sir. You'd better lose weight as fast as you can. Pay attention to your blood pressure."

Bill laughed, but be grudgingly, "It is too late for me to lose weight, I'm afraid. I have to work with my drawings long hours in my seats."

"It is never too late to lose weight!" The doctor tried to

encourage him, "You'll make it!"

"Are you serious, doctor? It's never too late to lose weight? " Bill asked.

"Yes! You could cheer up, sir." Doctor replied.

"It is never too late, so it should be too early for me to lose weight! Thank you, doctor!" Bill said happily and left the hospital.

Ⅱ. Find out your unknown words and phrases, write down and look up them.

Words	Meanings

Ⅲ. EXERCISES.

Reading Comprehension

1. According the doctor's advice, which of the following statements is true?

   A. Bill should work for long hours in seat.

   B. Bill should not take any exercise.

   C. Bill could stay up late.

   D. Bill needs to pay attention to his blood pressure.

2. What is the meaning of "the chair is the killer"?

   A. Sitting for a long time is harmful to health. B. The chair will beat Bill.

   C. The killer always sits on the chair. D. The chair is unhealthy.

3. Why doctor said "It is never too late to lose weight"?

   A. Because doctor wants to encourage Bill to lose weight.

   B. Because it is too early for Bill to lose weight.

   C. Because doctor believes Bill can lose weight naturally.

   D. Because Bill understands the real meaning.

Structure

4. I am so nervous, because I am quite ______ this conversation.

   A. happy for B. stressed for

   C. excited about D. street for

5. Skipping meals or eating very little can ______ kids.

   A. be beneficial to B. be good for

   C. be helpful to D. be harmful to

6. ______ every muscle in your body from head to toe. If you find any tense muscle, relax it.
   A. Pay to B. Pay respect to
   C. Pay attention to D. Pay attention for
7. It is never ______ late ______ lose weight.
   A. to...too B. so...as C. as...as D. too...to

Vocabulary

8. "The overweight man has to eat less sugar." Which one can replace "overweight" in this sentence?
   A. obese B. overload
   C. skinny D. health
9. "Are you serious, doctor? " In this passage, "serious" means ______ .
   A. the problem is really as bad as you say B. the doctor is qualified
   C. being overweight is bad for health D. telling the truth
10. Bill laughs, but grudgingly. It means Bill was ______ .
   A. happy B. worried C. unwilling D. thankful

GRAMMAR FOCUS

1．What should I do before the operation? 在手术前我应该做什么？

What should I...? 可用于询问他人的建议，表示“我应该怎么做”。

eg. What should I pay attention to? 我应该注意些什么？

2．Do you have any other advice/suggestion? 你还有其他的建议吗？

3．What about my diet today? 我今天的饮食要怎样呢？

What about / How about... 表示“(对于)……怎么样”，可用于询问他人对某事的意见和建议。

4．Would you please give me some suggestions? 能请你给我一些建议吗？

Would you please... 用于婉转客气地向他人询问建议。

5．给出建议的方式：you should/ you must/ you need to/ you could/ you'd better, etc.

eg. ① You should eat fluids. 你应该吃流食。

② You'd better sleep in supine position in the first 6 hours after the surgery．手术后的六小时，你最好保持仰卧姿势。

Section B Extensive Reading

Ⅰ. Read the passage. Tell how to nurse a woman after caesarean section.

The First Six Weeks after Caesarean Section

A caesarean section is a surgical procedure in which a baby is born through a cut made in the mother's abdominal wall and uterus. After a caesarean section, women usually stay in hospital for about three to five days. After the first week, the mother can go back home. There are tips to nurse her after the section in the first six weeks:

Let her get as much rest as she can.

Do not let her lift any weight that is heavier than the baby. Be careful of her back when she lifts.

Encourage her to take a gentle walk every day. This can have physical and emotional health benefits.

Help her take some pelvic floor exercises. She needs to be told that, her lower abdominal muscles and pelvic floor muscles will have weakened after pregnancy, and need strengthening.

Let her eat a healthy, high-fiber diet and drink plenty of water. Do this every day to avoid constipation.

Keep her wound clean and dry. Look for signs of infection (such as redness, pain, swelling of the wound or bad-smelling discharge).

She needs to be told that the loose clothing is allowable. And someone prefers firm, high-waisted compression underwear or control briefs to offer abdominal support, which can reduce pain and be worn for comfort for the first six weeks.

Looking after a new baby is hard for all women, but it can be harder for women when they are recovering from a caesarean. The key of the nursing is that the mother must be kind to herself.

Ⅱ. Find out your unknown words and phrases in the text, write down and look up them.

Words	Meanings

Ⅲ. According to the passage, fill T for true or F for false.

1. _______ The mother should not lift her baby.
2. _______ Some gentle walks are beneficial to the mother's physical and emotional health.
3. _______ Let her eat a healthy, high-fat diet every day to avoid constipation.
4. _______ It is necessary for keeping her wound clean and dry.
5. _______ The mother needs to know that the loose clothing and high-waisted compression underwear are all allowed.

Ⅳ. Discussion.

Can you name some special care for the baby after a caesarean section?

Section C Writing

Cover Letter 求职信

在求职时，仅凭简历就获得面试机会并非易事。因为简历通常只能罗列个人信息，内容常常单薄且缺乏生气。为了弥补简历的这一不足之处，求职者在投递简历的同时，附上一封 Cover Letter，即求职信，不仅能增强求职竞争力，还能显示出求职者应聘的诚意与端正的态度。

SAMPLE

The following is a cover letter. Please read and try to understand it.

Dear Ms. Rose,

Please accept my application for the position of nurse, advertised in the *China Daily*.

I have always enjoyed working on nursing. I have worked as a nutrition nurse at ZA hospital. I gained a lot of experience there, such as elderly care and surgical nursing, which I think would be valuable to your hospital.

I have enclosed my resume, and I would very much like to talk with you in your hospital.

I look forward to hearing from you.

Yours truly,

Jane

KNOWLEDGE

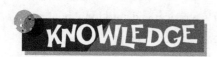

求职信的正文内容一般分为三部分：

1. 写明应聘职位

正文首先应叙述一下你是从何渠道得知招聘消息的，并写明你打算应聘的是哪一个职位。

2. 简述经历特色

正文第二部分简述自己的工作经历，重点阐述与应聘岗位最相关的经历。同时，可说明应聘单位为什么吸引你，你又能做出什么贡献。

3. 提出面试请求

可以首先感谢阅信人花时间读了你的信，随后提出请求，请阅信人给你一个面试的机会。

EXERCISES

Fill in the following cover letter.

1.__________________, (尊敬的王先生)

In response to a 2.__________________(招聘广告) in newspaper of April 15th, I wish to apply for the position of nurse.

I am 20 years old and 3.__________________(我将从护理学校毕业). I have some experience in nursing, 4.__________________(我曾在第一医院做实习护士) for 10 months.

My resume, 5.__________________(毕业证复印件) and my photo are enclosed for your reference. I believe they may be found satisfactory.

I shall be obligated if you will give me a personal interview at your convenience.

6.__________________(盼早日回复).

Very truly yours,

Zeng Li

Unit 10

Rehabilitation Instruction

Section A *All You Need to Do is to Spend Less Time Surfing the Internet.*

Language Goals: Talk about Some Medical Equipments for Rehabilitation and Express Rehabilitation Care in English.

WARM-UP

I. Match the phrases with pictures.

________ walker

________ removable denture

________ artificial limb

________ wheelchair

________ hand gripper

________ hearing-aid

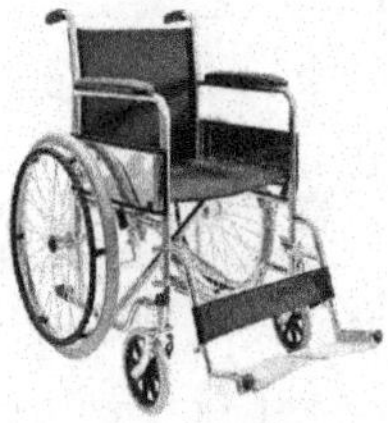

A

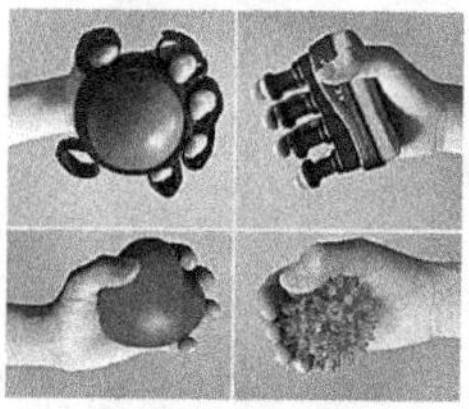

B

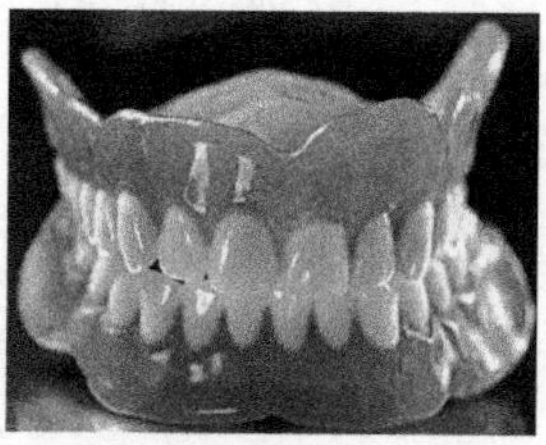

C

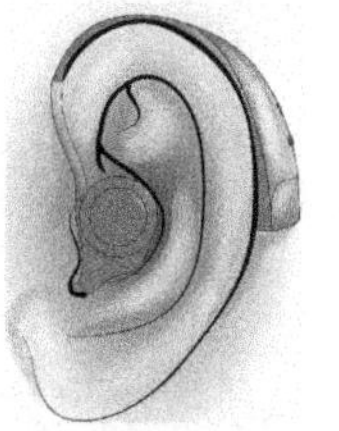

D

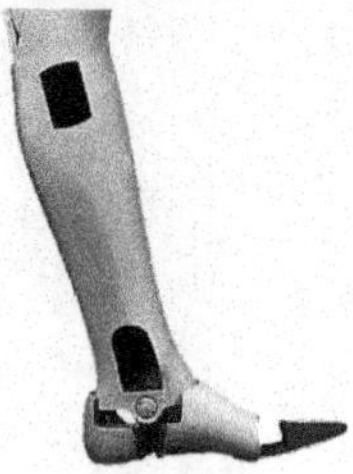

E

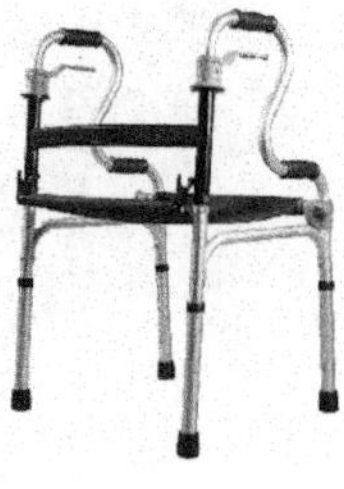

F

Ⅱ. Listen and number the pictures 1 to 4 in the order you hear them.

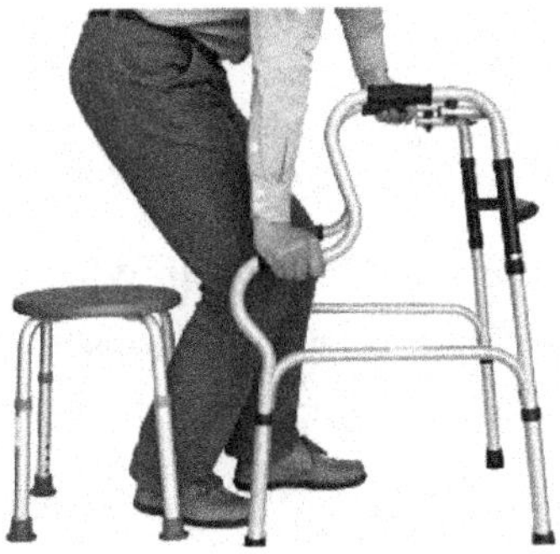

_______ practice walking

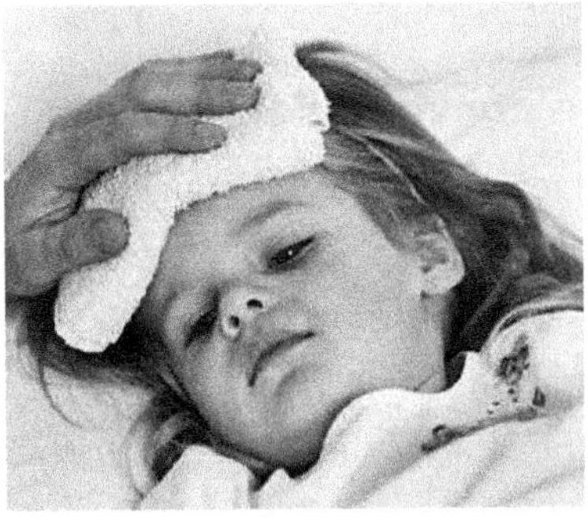

_______ use physical cooling

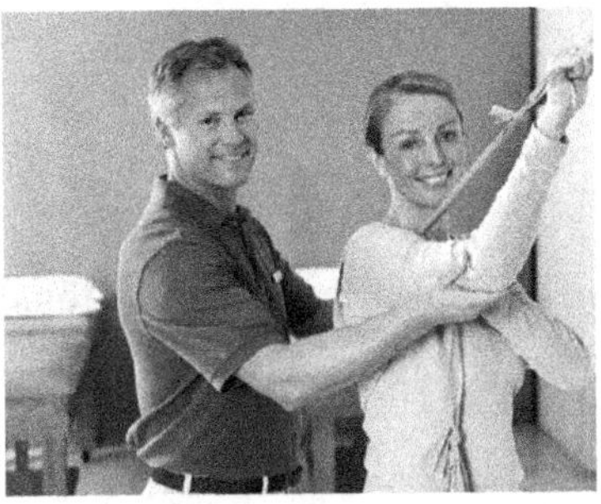

_______ do physical training

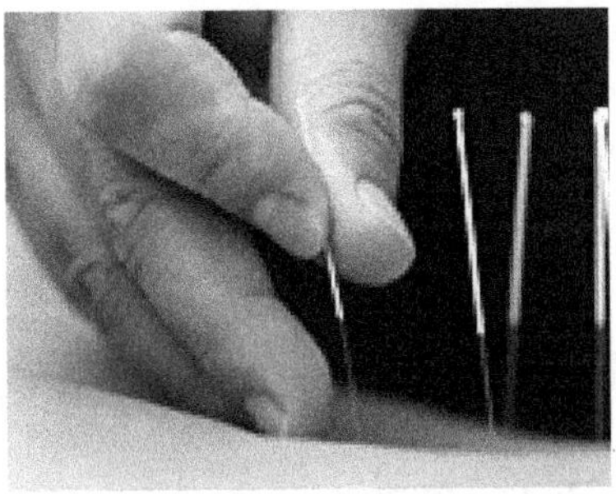

_______ give acupuncture

Ⅲ. Listen again and match the person with what they are doing now.

Bob's grandfather	is practicing walking with a walker.
Mr. Mark	is helping his wife with physical training.
Mary's mother	is cooling Mary's head with a cold towel.
Mr. Black	is giving acupuncture a whirl.

Ⅳ. Listen and read.

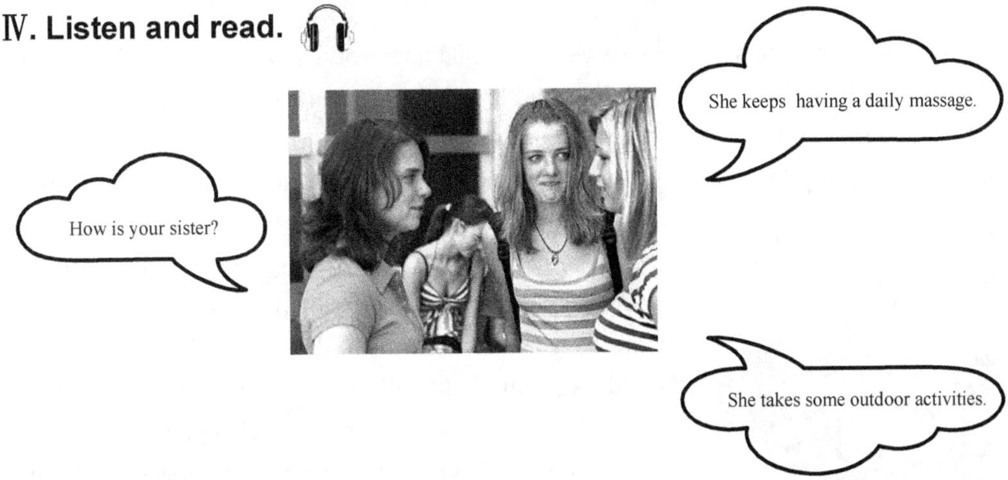
How is your sister?
She keeps having a daily massage.
She takes some outdoor activities.

DIALOGUE

Role-play the conversation.

John: Good morning, Mike, long time no see.

Mike: Oh, morning, John, long time no see. Wow, you don't look well. What is wrong?

John: These days, I surf too much on the Internet. I feel pain in my eyes and shoulders, and I have trouble falling asleep.

Mike: That is bad. You should spend less time surfing the Internet. Do you have any other hobbies?

John: Mm, I like reading when I am free.

Mike: You should take some outdoor activities, such as jogging and swimming.

John: But I am not interested in jogging and swimming.

Mike: What about playing basketball?

John: Oh, yes, I love it.

Mike: Well, we'll have a basketball game with Dongfang Health School tomorrow. Will you come and join us?

John: That's great. I bet we'll win.

Mike: Sure. See you tomorrow, then.

John: See you.

READING

Ⅰ. Read the passage and know about the work of rehabilitation nurse.

The Dream of a Rehabilitation Nurse

Lily graduated from a nursing school 5 years ago, and now works as a nurse in a rehabilitation center. Every day, she gives patients injections and dressings. She massages them and helps them with rehabilitation trainings.

Now Lily is helping Mr. Wang with a ball to carry out rehabilitation training of hand functions. Lily has Mr. Wang hold the ball in one hand, slowly raise the arm, fold the fingers and grasp the ball. More than 20 days ago, Mr. Wang was hospitalized with an intracerebral haemorrhage which led to the left limb dysfunction. After these days' training, Mr. Wang can grab the ball without falling. This makes the family members feel hopeful.

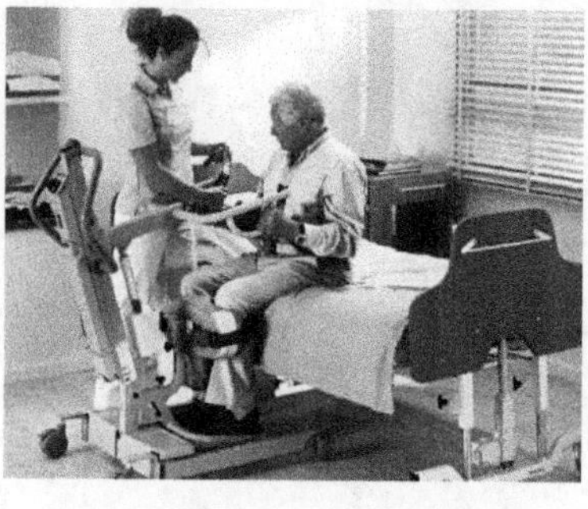

Mrs. Liu, a lady in sixties, suffered from a cerebral infarction and is getting treatment at the hospital. She could barely move a finger when admitted. For more than a month, Lily has kept giving her a daily massage and turn-over practice. Now the old lady can walk slowly by holding the wall.

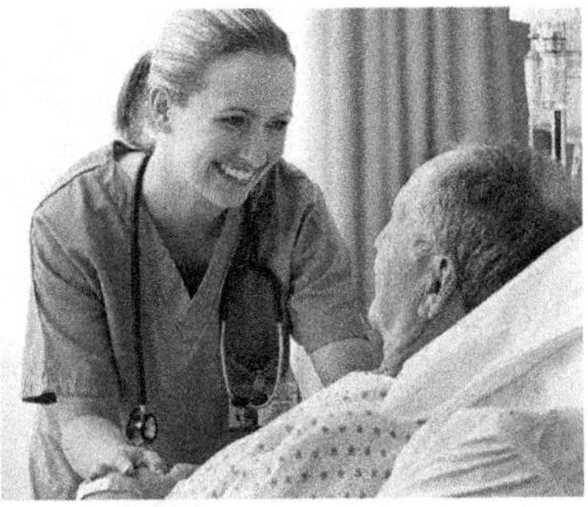

There are many more cases like these. Seeing these patients gradually recover, Lily thinks that her efforts are worth it. No matter how tired she feels, she will stick to her job. It is her greatest wish to see the patients restart a healthy and happy life.

Ⅱ. Find out your unknown words and phrases, write down and look up them.

Words	Meanings

Ⅲ. EXERCISES.

Reading Comprehension

1. Lily is a nurse who works in the ______.
   A. inpatient department　　B. rehabilitation center
   C. department of general surgery　　D. pharmacy
2. Lily is helping Mr. Wang with______to carry out rehabilitationtraining of hand functions.
   A. a bowl　　B. a pen　　C. a ball　　D. an apple
3. Mr. Wang suffered from ______.
   A. an intracerebral haemorrhage　　B. toothache
   C. a cerebral infarction　　D. a cold
4. Mrs. Liu suffered from ______.
   A. an intracerebral haemorrhage　　B. toothache
   C. a cerebral infarction　　D. a cold
5. Lily's dream is ______.
   A. to be a doctor
   B. to be a head nurse
   C. to do some operations herself
   D. to make her patients restart a healthy and happy life

Vocabulary & Structure

6. Lily graduated ______a nursing school 5 years ago, and now works as a nurse in a

rehabilitation center.

A. at B. off C. of D. from

7. Mr. Wang______with an intracerebral haemorrhage.

A. hospital B. was hospital

C. hospitalized D. was hospitalized

8. Mrs. Liu could______move a finger when ______.

A. barely,admitted B. barely,suffered

C. nearly,admitted D. nearly,suffered

9. Lily has kept ______Mrs. Liu a daily massage and turn-over practice for more than a month.

A. give B. gives C. giving D. given

10. No matter______tired Lily feels, she will stick to her job.

A. how B. what C. when D. where

GRAMMAR FOCUS

1. Long time no see. 很久不见。

2. I feel pain in my eyes and shoulders, and I have trouble falling asleep. 我眼睛和肩膀疼，并且入睡困难。

3. — Do you have any other hobbies? 您有其他爱好吗？

— Mm, I like reading when I am free. 嗯，有空时我喜欢阅读。

4. You should take some outdoor activities, such as jogging. 您应该从事一些户外活动，例如慢跑。

5. But I am not interested in jogging and swimming. 但我不喜欢慢跑和游泳。

Section B Extensive Reading

I. Read the passage and know about the rehabilitation care.

Any Ideas of Rehabilitation Care?

Many people have few ideas about rehabilitation. Many patients with diseases such as spinal cord injury, stroke and cerebral palsy will recuperate at home after surgery. Most of their families think that they will recover quickly. But actually, some of them will be confined to bed forever.

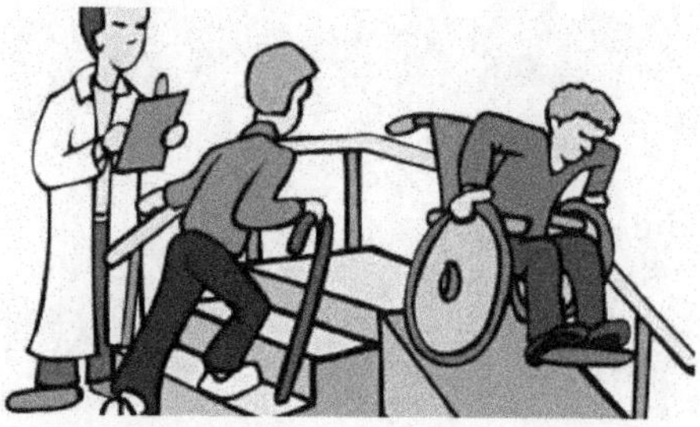

Successful rehabilitation can help these patients recover to an ideal health level or even help them regain their working ability. It's a pity that some families are unable to provide good family care for quick recovery. Some patients' health condition becomes worse because they don't get enough rehabilitation care from their families. It has been proved that with good family care more than half of the stroke patients can regain the self-care ability after about one year's valid rehabilitation care, while only 5% are in full need of help.

Ⅱ. Find out your unknown words and phrases in the text, write down and look up them.

Words	Meanings

Ⅲ. According to the passage, fill T for true or F for false.

1. ______ All the patients will have complete recovery after surgery.
2. ______ Some patients will be confined to bed forever.
3. ______ Patients' health condition will be better after the subsequent attacks of stroke.
4. ______ More than half of the stroke patients can regain the self-care ability after about one year's valid rehabilitation care.
5. ______ One of rehabilitation care's responsibilities is to strengthen patients'existing functions.

Section C Writing

Resume

求职简历是求职者对自己过往工作、学习和生活经历的简要概述，常用表格的形式表示。

SAMPLE

The following is the resume of a student who will graduate from a health school this year. Please read and try to understand it.

PERSONAL DATA					
Name	Meilin Yang	Gender	Female	Date of Birth	Feb.2nd,1999
Height	165cm	Weight	53kg	Health	Excellent
Address	375 Antu Road Shanghai, 200000	Tel.	021-637563××	E-mail	Meilin@163.com

JOB OBJECTIVE	To be employed by a hospital in Shanghai as a nurse.
Education	Nursing major, ×××Health School, 2014,Sept.—2017,May.; ×××Middle School, 2011, Sept.—2014. May.
Skills	1. Have a good command of both spoken and written English; 2. Be skilled in use of Windows/Office/FoxPro.
Scholarships & Awards	1. The Second Prize of the National Nursing Skills Contest for Secondary Vocational Group 2017. May.; 2. First-class Scholarship 2015.Sept.—2016. Sept.; 3. Third-class Scholarship 2014. Sept.—2015. Sept.
Qualifications	Registering License for Nurses to Practice in the People's Republic of China
Activities	1. Having internship at the No.1 People's Hospital 2016. Sept.—2017. Apr.; 2. Volunteering at the welfare institutions 2016. July.—2016. Aug.
Hobbies	swimming & singing

KNOWLEDGE

完整的简历一般包括以下内容：

1. Personal Data：个人资料

个人资料包含姓名、性别、出生日期、身高、体重、健康状况、地址、电话号码、电子邮箱等。个人资料中可以附上一张近照，给招聘单位留下初步印象。

2. Job Objective：求职目标

简历中应直接写明希望应聘的职位，给人以目标明确的感觉。

3. Education：教育经历

简历常使用倒叙的方式，把曾经就读的学校名称、时间、所学专业和取得的学位等信息一一列举。

4. Work Experience：工作经历

简历常使用倒叙的方式，列举曾经就职的工作单位名称、职位和工作时间等。

5. Awards：奖励

简历应列出学习、工作中获得的各种奖励。

6. Social Activities：社会活动

这部分内容对于没有工作经历的学生尤为重要，它在一定程度上反映出应聘者的工作热情和态度以及人际沟通能力，加深用人单位对求职者的印象。

7. Hobbies/Specialties：个人爱好或特长

个人爱好和特长应在简历中有所体现。

EXERCISE

Fill in the following form with your own information.

PERSONAL DATA					
Name		Gender		Date of Birth	
Height		Weight		Health	
Address		Tel.		E-mail	

JOB OBJECTIVE	
Education	
Skills	
Scholarships & Awards	
Qualifications	
Activities	
Hobbies	

参 考 文 献

李正亚，2012．全国医护英语水平考试（护理类）应考大全．上海：上海外语教育出版社

马丽娃，杨蓉，2006．临床医学英语．北京：中国科技技术出版社

宋军，2006．护理专业英语．北京：人民卫生出版社

汤先觉，2009. 英语．北京：人民卫生出版社

唐巧英，2009．医护英语．北京：外语教学与研究出版社

唐巧英，2013．医护英语．北京：外语教学与研究出版社

唐巧英，2015．医护英语．北京：外语教学与研究出版社

陶三琴，冯欣，2015．英语．北京：人民卫生出版社

徐小贞，2015．新职业英语（行业篇 - 医护英语）. 第 2 版．北京：外语教学与研究出版社

王洵，2011. 实用护理英语．南京：南京大学出版社

王文秀，2010．英汉对照医务英语会话．北京：人民卫生出版社

王守仁，2013．实用综合教程．上海：上海外语教育出版社

Judith Perry，蔡碧华，沈宁，2006．护理美语．北京：科学出版社

Virginia Allum, Patricia McGarr, 2010．护理英语 1（Cambridge English for Nursing）. 北京：中国青年出版社

课 文 注 释

Unit 1

Section A

1．She is working for a big hospital. 她在一家大医院上班。

现在进行时：is/are/am+doing（动词的进行式）...

表示当前正在进行的状态、动作。例：

Listen. She is singing an English song. 听，她正在唱一首英文歌。

2．Being a nurse is her dream．成为一名护士是她的梦想。

Being a nurse 是动名词，作句子的主语。例：

Swimming is good for health. 游泳有益健康。

3．She has worked in this big hospital for over 20 years. 她已经在这所大医院工作了二十多年。

现在完成时：have/has+done（动词的完成式）...

(1) 表示过去发生的动作对现在造成的影响或结果；

(2) 表示过去的动作或状态持续到现在。例：

I have lost my pen. 我的钢笔丢了。

4．She must be at least forty years old. 她肯定至少有四十岁了。

情态动词 +do（动词原型）...

情态动词用在行为动词前，表示说话人对这一动作或状态的看法或主观设想。情态动词虽然数量不多，但用途广泛，主要有：can (could), may (might), must, need, ought to, dare (dared), shall (should), will (would) must not. 例：

You may drive the car. 你可以开这辆车。

Section B

1．She could have lived an easy, comfortable life. But instead she chose to work hard and care for the sick. 她本可以拥有轻松舒适的生活，但却选择了辛勤工作、照顾病患。

instead / instead of 表示“反而；代替”。例：

Take a shower instead of a bath. 洗淋浴吧，别用浴缸了。

2．Florence Nightingale was one of the world’s great nurses. 弗洛伦斯·南丁格尔是世界上伟大的护士之一。

one of the sths. / sbs.（名词的复数形式）表示“……之一”。例：

She is one of fair-minded people I know. 她是我所认识的极公正的人之一。

3. ...they thought it would be better if she didn’t work. 他们认为女儿成为一名家庭主妇会更好。

It would be better if sb. did sth. 虚拟语气，表示“假如……会更好”。例：

It would be better if you had sports every day. 如果你每天运动会更好。

4．Nurses were not well respected at the time. 在那时，护士这个职业并不被尊重。

被动语态：be 动词 +done（动词的完成式）。例：

We believe him. 我们相信他。=He is believed by us. 他被我们相信。

Unit 2

Section A

1．Doctor Sherry Brain works at the school clinic. 雪莉・布莱恩医生在这家校园诊所工作。

sb. works at/in... 是介绍某人在某处工作的常用句型。介词 at 与 in 的不同用法需要注意：at... 多用于指较小的地点、场所，即在具体某一位置；而 in... 多用于指较大的地方，表示空间或范围。例：

We live at No. 87, Beijing Road. 我们住在北京路 87 号。

She works in a hospital. 她在一家医院里上班。

2．It was a cold day, but she was in a very short skirt. 这一天很寒冷，但她只穿了一条很短的裙子。

in 作为介词时，可表示"穿着、戴着、带着"。具体用法为：in+ 衣服 / 颜色。例：

the woman in white 穿白衣服的女子；the man in the blue suit 穿蓝色西装的男子。

3．She told the doctor that she felt headache. 她告诉医生她感到头疼。

本句是由 that 引导的宾语从句。通常在 say, think, wish , hope, tell, see, believe, agree, expect, hear, feel 等动词后加 that，引出宾语从句。宾语从句只可使用陈述语序，即"引导词 + 主语 + 谓语 + 宾语 + 其他"。宾语从句的时态受主句限制，主句是一般过去时态，从句必须用相应的表示过去的时态。特别需要注意的是，表示"建议"（ advise, suggest, propose, recommend ）后的宾语从句，从句谓语应由"should+ 动词原形"构成。课文中多次出现宾语从句：

(1) Dr. Sherry told her that she had caught a cold and it was not serious. 雪莉医生告诉她，她感冒了，并不严重。

(2) Dr. Sherry advised that she should take the pills three times a day for 3 days and remember to wear warmer clothes on cold days. 雪莉医生建议她每天服药三次，坚持 3 天。在寒冷的天气里要记得穿暖和些的衣服。

(3) She said that she had a stomachache. 她说她肚子痛。

(4) Sara said that she had 4 big hamburgers, a large Coca-Cola with ice as well as a large box of ice-cream. 萨拉说她吃了四个大汉堡，一大杯加冰的可口可乐，外加一大盒冰激凌。

4．What a huge lunch! 这顿午餐真是太丰盛了！

What a busy afternoon! 多么忙碌的一下午啊！

这是由 what 引导的感叹句，what 意为"多么"，修饰名词（被强调部分）。由 what 引导的感叹句，主要用来修饰名词，分为三种结构：

(1) What+a/an+ 形容词 + 可数名词单数 + 主语 + 谓语 +! 例：

What a cute boy he is! 多么可爱的小男孩啊！

(2) What+ 形容词 + 可数名词复数 + 主语 + 谓语 + ！ 例：

What warm-hearted children they are! 他们是多么热心的孩子啊！

(3) What+ 形容词 + 不可数名词 + 主语 + 谓语 +! 例：

What pleasant weather it is! 多么宜人的天气啊！

Section B

1. Hospitals are the places for the treatment and care of people who are ill or sick or who need a doctor, for example, in pregnancy. 医院是给病人或者需要看医生的人，提供治疗和护理的地方如孕妇。

本句中的两个 who 为引导词，引导出的定语从句修饰 people。be ill/sick 表示“生病了”；be in pregnancy 则表示“怀孕，妊娠期”。

2. Hospitals may be divided into general hospitals and special hospitals. 医院可以分为综合性医院和专科医院。

本句中 be divided into 使用了被动语态，翻译为“被分为……”

英语动词有两种语态：主动语态和被动语态。主动语态表示主语是动作的执行者，被动语态表示主语是动作的承受者。汉语中常用“被”“给”“由”“受”等词表示被动，而英语则由“助动词 be+ 及物动词的过去分词”构成被动语态。

3. Patients of all ages and with different illnesses and injuries can be treated in the general hospitals. 不同年龄段的病人和不同伤病的患者都可以在综合性医院进行治疗。

本句中 of all ages 以及 with different illnesses and injuries 是介词短语做后置定语，修饰 patients。其中，Patients of all ages 译为“不同年龄段的病人”，而 patients with different illnesses and injuries 译为“不同伤病的患者”。

4. Doctors, nurses and other medical workers make up the staff of a hospital. 医院的工作人员由医生、护士和其他医务人员组成。

make up 表示“构成，组成”。例：

The committee is made up of six women. 委员会由六位妇女组成。

Unit 3

Section A

1. in order not to influence the next work... 为了不影响接下来的工作……

in order to 后面直接接动词原形，表示“为了……, 以便……”，其否定形式为 in order not to，例：

In order not to wake the baby we went in quietly. 为了不惊醒小孩，我们轻轻地走了进去。

2. I couldn't help asking. 我忍不住问了一句。

could not help doing sth. 表示“不得不、禁不住做某事”。例：

She couldn't help smiling. 她禁不住笑了起来。

3. 美国人和中国人对楼层的表述方式是一致的，除了地下室，地面楼层叫做一楼，依次往上是二楼、三楼……但英国人表述楼层的方式是不一样的，英国人把一层称为 the ground floor，二层称为 the first floor，依次类推。即英国人告诉你 the second floor，其实是我们常说的三楼。

当表述“医院的二楼有一个灭火器时”：

英国人这样说：There is a fire extinguisher on the first floor of the hospital.

美国人这样说：There is a fire extinguisher on the second floor of the hospital.

Section B

1. Just then five bodies showed up at my desk, a pale woman and four small children. 就在这时，五个人出现在我的办公桌前：一个面色苍白的妇女和四个小孩儿。

show up 表示“显而易见，到场，出现”。例：

He showed up an hour late. 他来了，迟到了一小时。

2. Something was wrong, I didn't say anything but explained that it might be a little while before a doctor saw her. 事情有点不对头，但是我也没说什么，只是解释说医生要过一阵儿才会来给她检查。

句中的 that 在动词 explain 后，引导宾语从句。大多数动词都可以带宾语从句，that 后面需要跟一个完整的句子。例：

We know that we should study hard. 我们知道我们应该努力学习。

I expect that they will win. 我预料到他们会赢。

3. No address — they were homeless. 上面没写地址——他们无家可归。

-less 是一个形容词性的后缀，表示“无，不做，不能”。例：

care→careless 粗心的；use→useless 无用的；name→nameless 无名的；price→priceless 无价的.

4. As seriously as we met the physical needs of the patients, our team worked to meet the needs of a family who just wanted to be warm on Christmas. 我们的团队工作严肃，就像满足当天其他患者的需要一样，我们尽力满足这家人只想过一个温暖圣诞节的愿望。

(1) as...as 用于比较句型，中间插入的是形容词或副词的原级，意思是“达到与……相同的程度”。本句中的 seriously 为副词，意为“严肃地；认真地”。

as long as “长达……之久”；as much as “高达……；与……一样多”。

(2) 句中的 who 引导定语从句，先行词为 family，指“一家人”。

Unit 4

Section A

1. I have been working in the hospital as a practice nurse for one month. 我已经在医院做了一个月实习护士。

现在完成进行时：has / have been+doing（动词的进行式）...

表示动作从某一时间开始，一直持续到现在，或者刚刚终止，或者可能仍然要继续下去。例：

She has been playing tennis since she was eight. 她从八岁起就在打网球。

2. When I was ill, I have been given several injections... 当我病了时，我打过几次针。

现在完成时的被动语态：has / have been done（动词的过去分词）...

表示过去的动作对现在造成的影响或结果，但主语为动作的承受者，即“已经被……”。例：

His bike has been repaired. 他的自行车已经被修好了。

3. After washing my hands carefully, I met my patient who needed a penicillin injection. 仔细清洁双手后，我见到了我的病人，她需要注射盘尼西林。

After+doing 短语为句子的时间状语，表示“在……之后”。例：

After having lunch, Tom took a rest. 午餐后，汤姆休息了一下。

Section B

1. Intravenous (IV) infusions are one of the most important treatments in hospital nowadays. 静脉输液是如今医院最重要的治疗手段之一。

one of the most... 表示“最……的之一”。例：

Football is one of the most popular sports. 足球是最流行的运动之一。

2. Intravenous infusions are commonly referred to as drips. 静脉输液通常称为点滴。

refer to as... 表示“把……称作……”。例：

All his classmates referred to him as “Clever Boy”. 他的同学都叫他聪明男孩。

3. IV infusion of drugs is normally given to patients who cannot be treated orally or by injection. 静脉输液给药通常适用于不能口服或者注射治疗的病人。

句中 who 引导定语从句，修饰 patients。例：

The boy who is singing is my friend. 正在唱歌的那个男孩是我的朋友。

4. The fluids cannot drip too quickly and must be given slowly in order not to overload the patient. 液体不能滴太快，必须慢点儿滴，以免病人负荷不了。

情态动词被动语态：must be+done（动词的完成式）... 例：

The work must be finished today. 工作必须今天完成。

Unit 5

Section A

1. At first, he sold bottles of a cure for colds for just a dollar a bottle. 开始的时候他卖的只是一美元一瓶的感冒药。

cure 作名词，表示“治疗……的药物”。例：

cure for headache 治疗头痛的药。

2. “And now, ladies and gentlemen,” he shouted, “here is the medicine you have been waiting for.” 他大声说道：“先生们，女士们，这就是你们一直等着的药。”

现在完成进行时：have been doing... 例：

I have been learning English since 3 years ago. 我从三年前就一直学习英语了。（还会继续学习下去。）

3. Another person cried, “Yes, you look as if you were at least sixty years old.” 另一个人大喊道：“是的，你看起来至少有六十岁了。”

as if 表示“似乎；好像”。例：

They looked as if they hadn’t washed in days. 他们看起来好像已经有好些天没洗澡了。

Section B

1. So far, they have tested it only in laboratory animals. 到目前为止，他们只在实验室动物身上进行了测试。

so far 表示“到目前为止”。例：

So far, 57 students have taken the test. 到目前为止，有 57 个学生参加了测试。

2. The team says that the treatment killed the cancer and avoided healthy cells better than other treatments. 研究小组说，这种治疗相比其他方法，能更好地杀死癌细胞并避开健康细胞。

better than 表示“比……更好；优于……”。例：

After all, 15 minutes of exercise is better than nothing. 毕竟，锻炼 15 分钟比不锻炼好。

3. In this study, they say that eighty percent of the mice treated with the nano-cells lived more than sixty-five days. 在这项研究中，他们说用纳米细胞治疗的老鼠中有百分之八十的寿命超过六十五天。

...percent of... 表示“……的百分之……”。例：

Almost 80 percent of the city's residents were born elsewhere. 这座城市有 80% 的居民出生于异地。

Unit 6

Section A

1. A medical examination is used to check your overall health. 体格检查用于检查你身体的总体健康情况。

一般现在时的用法：

(1) 表示现在的状态、能力、性格等。例：

He works in a hospital. 他在医院工作。

I can speak English. 我会说英语。

I am creative and outgoing. 我富有创造力，并且性格外向。

(2) 表示经常或习惯性的动作，常与频率副词连用。例：

She goes to school every day. 她每天去上学。

My grandma often goes to the part on Sundays. 我的奶奶周日经常去公园。

(3) 表示客观真理或科学事实。例：

The moon goes around the earth. 月亮绕着地球转。

Two plus one is three. 二加一等于三。

2. It examines many organs and other parts of the body, such as heart, lung, eyesight, stomach and so on. 它能检查身体的很多器官和其他部位，例如心脏、肺部、视力，胃等。

such as 和 for example 都可以用来列举，但两者之间有以下区别：

	辨析	例句
such as	用于列举事物，常放在所列举的名词前面，但列举的只是前面所提内容的一部分	I like many colors, such as blue, red and yellow. 我喜欢很多种颜色，例如蓝色、红色和黄色。
for example	用于举例说明某现象，可用于句首、句中或句末，需用逗号隔开	You should live a healthy lifestyle, for example, you should do some sports every day. 你要养成良好的生活习惯，比如每天去运动。

3. Both telephone appointment and online booking are wildly used in daily life. 在日常生活中，电话预约和网上预约都非常流行。

both...and... 表示“……和……”，谓语使用复数，否定形式为 neither...nor...，但其谓语的单复数应遵循就近原则。例：

Both he and I are in Grade 1. 我和他都在一年级。

Neither he nor I am from Shenzhen. 我和他都不是来自深圳。

4. During the exam, be honest to your doctor. Make sure you speak up with any questions or concerns you have about your health, no matter how minor they may seem. 在体检过程中，请诚实地面对医生，确保你毫无保留地说出关于你健康的问题或担心，即便是很小的一点也不例外。

"no matter+ 疑问词" 引导让步状语从句。例：

No matter how busy I am, I always try to read books. 无论多忙，我总会设法看书。

Section B

1. If you plan to visit Canada for six months or less, a medical exam is not required. 如果你打算去加拿大的时间在六个月以内，你不需要体检。

句中的 a medical exam is not required 为被动语态。被动语态表示主语是动作的承受者，其基本句型是："主语 +be+ 动词的过去分词"。

以下三种情况中经常使用被动语态：

（1）不知道或没必要指出动作的执行者。例：

My bag was stolen yesterday. 我的书包昨天被偷了。

The book is written for children. 这本书是为儿童所写的。

（2）强调动作的承受者。例：

The glass is broken by John. 玻璃被约翰打碎了。

（3）出于礼貌而避免提到动作的执行者。例：

He was asked to give a speech at the meeting. 他被要求在会议上发言。

2. There are other situations where you also need to have this exam. 还有其他一些情况，你也必须体检。

当先行词为具有地点意义的词，如 place, situation, stage 等时，关系副词可使用 where。例：

I often go to the place where we used to see a film. 我经常去我们之前看电影的地方。

3. However, not all the doctors can perform the medical exam. You must see a doctor on the certain list of panel physicians. 然而，并不是所有的医生都能进行体检，你必须找到名单上专门的体检机构，他们会给你做完整的体格检查。

英语中常用的几种关联词有：

（1）表示转折：however, but。例：

She was born in China. However, she cannot speak Chinese. 她虽然在中国出生，但她不会说中文。

He feels tired, but he doesn't want to go to bed. 他感觉很累，但不想上床休息。

（2）表示并列：and, also。例：

He is a teacher, and he sings very well. 他是一名老师，并且唱歌非常好听。

I want to go shopping. My mother also wants to come with me. 我想去购物，我妈妈也想和我一起去。

（3）表示递进：what's more; moreover。例：

The skirt fits you well. What's more, it's very cheap. 这条裙子很适合你，并且它很便宜。

She is a beautiful girl. Moreover, she likes helping others. 她是个漂亮的女孩。更重要的是，她乐于助人。

（4）表示让步：although。例：

She seemed a baby although she was already thirty. 尽管她已经三十岁了，看上去还像个小孩。

Unit 7

Section A

1．When I'm feeling ill or sick, I will go to the hospital to have a regular check-up in the outpatient department. 当我感到难受或生病时，我会去医院门诊做一个定期检查。

(1) feel 作为感官动词，表示人的感觉，后面可接形容词。例：

I'm feeling ill or sick. 我感到难受 / 我生病了。

I don't feel very well today. 我今天感到不太舒服。

(2) have a regular check-up 表示“定期检查”。

check up 作为动词短语，有体格检查、检查身体之意；check-up 作为名词，表示“体检、检查身体”，如 a routine check-up（常规体检）的复数形式为 check-ups。

(3) in the outpatient department 在门诊；in the inpatient department 在住院部。

2．After registration, I complained of having been vomiting for three days. 在挂号处，我主诉已经吐了三天。

(1) registration 作名词，表示“挂号、注册、登记”；registration office（挂号处），online registration（网上挂号）；register 作为动词，表示“注册、登记”。

(2) complain of 作为动词短语，表示“抱怨、诉苦、主诉、患者描述症状”等。例：

They may complain of diarrhea。他们可能会主诉腹泻。

Nurses complain of being overworked and underpaid. 护士抱怨工作劳累过度而报酬过低。

What important news it is! 这是多么重要的消息啊！

3．I was asked to go through the admission procedure. 我被告知要经过住院流程。

(1) ask sb. to do sth. 表示“让某人做某事、要求某人做……”，本句中使用了被动语态结构，即 sb. was asked to do sth.

(2) go through 作为动词短语，表示“通过、完成、经历、经受”。例：

Go through the admission procedure. 办理住院手续。

He was going through a very difficult time. 他正处于非常艰难的时期。

4．After a while, the ward nurse came to ask me if I am allergic to any medication, for example, penicillin. 过了一会儿，病房护士来问我是否对药物过敏，例如青霉素。

(1) after a while 表示“不久、过了一会儿”；for a while 表示“暂时，一段时间”；in a while 则表示“在一段时间之内”，一般和将来时连用。

(2) be allergic to something 表示“对……过敏”。allergic 用作形容词，其名词为 allergy, 表示“过敏性反应”，可用于 Somebody has an allergy to something 的句型中，表示“某人对……过敏”。例：

She is allergic to penicillin. = She has an allergy to penicillin. 她对青霉素过敏。

5. She also reminded me that if I felt itchy or short of breath, just let her know at once. 她提醒我，如果我感到痒或呼吸短促，立即通知她。

(1)remind sb. that...；remind sb. of sth. 表示“提醒某人某事；使人想起某事，使人回忆

起某事”。例：

He reminds me of his father. 他让我想起他的父亲。

She reminded me that I hadn’t written to my mother. 她提醒了我，我还没有给妈妈写信。

(2) short of breath 表示“呼吸困难、喘不过气来、呼吸急促”。

Section B

1. The admission of a patient is a formal process of entry into the hospital. 病人的入院是进入医院的正规程序。

admission 作为名词，表示“入院、住院”，the admission of a patient 表示患者的住院、病人的入院，与 of a patient 结合构成名词短语，在句中作主语。

formal 作为形容词，表示“正规的”，a formal process 译为“正规流程、正规程序”；entry 作为名词，表示“进入、入场”，后面往往与介词 into 连接，表示“进入某场合”；entry into the hospital 表示“进入医院”。

2. What’s more, inpatients’data will be collected to assess the clinical condition and nursing needs during the process. 另外，这一过程也是为评估病人临床状况和护理需要而收集资料的一种方法。

What’s more 表示递进，译为“然而 / 还有……”，独立使用，more 后面不加词和句，往往以逗号隔开，既可以放句首，也可以放句中，放句首时 w 要大写。

英语动词有两种语态：主动语态和被动语态。主动语态表示主语是动作的执行者，被动语态表示主语是动作的承受者。被动语态也像主动语态一样有相应的时态。

本句中 data will be collected to 使用了被动语态将来时态，翻译为“数据将被收集起来……”

3. For the patients, admission card, admission form, ID card, National Health Insurance IC card and related certificates (major illness/injury card, etc.) as well as the previous medical records have to be checked when they are coming for admission. 对于患者来说，他们办理入院手续时，需要检查入院卡、入院申请表、身份证、国家医疗保险 IC 卡及相关证书（证明所患的主要疾病或严重伤的卡片等）以及以前的医疗记录。

本句中 be checked 使用了被动语态，在此不强调动作的发出者，只强调入院卡、入院申请表、身份证、国家医疗保险 IC 卡及相关证书（证明所患的主要疾病或严重伤的卡片等）这些物品入院前需要被检查。

admission 作为名词，表示“入院、住院”，因此 admission card 表示“入院卡”，admission form 表示“入院申请表”。admit 作为动词，表示准许入场（入会、入校、入院），在表示某人入住医院时往往使用被动语态。例：

She was admitted to the hospital. 她住院了。

4. As soon as the patient is admitted, the nurses should give him a physical examination. 病人一入院，护士就应该给他做体检。

as soon as 表示“一……就……”，引导时间状语从句且当主句用一般过去时时，从句用一般过去时或过去完成时。例：

I will tell him the news as soon as he comes back. 他一回来，我就把这个消息告诉他。

give sb. a physical examination 表示“给某人进行体检”，physical examination 表示“身体检查、健康检查”。

Unit 8

Section A

1. Before long, all necessary examinations were completed after the admission. 不久后，为李先生所做的一系列必要的入院检查就已全部完成。

现在时的被动语态：am/ is/ are+done（动词的过去分词）...

过去时的被动语态：was/ were+done（动词的过去分词）...

表示某一时间某件事情被完成，或某一事物被动承受某种行为动作。例：

The necessary measures were taken for Mr. Li during the hospitalization. 在李先生住院期间，一系列治疗措施都被用于对他的治疗。

2. during the hospitalization. 在生病住院期间。例：

During her hospitalization, Mrs. Jiang was looked after carefully by Mr. Jiang. 生病住院期间，江太太被江先生非常精心地照料着。

3. Measures for improving circulation, controlling blood pressure and improving mood and sleep were taken to Dr. Lu's instructions. 根据医嘱，针对改善血液循环、控制血压及改善情绪和睡眠等方面的措施被用在他的治疗上。

for... 表示"针对……而进行的，为了……而做的"；were taken... 为被动语态，表示"被使用"；to the doctor's instructions = according to the doctor's advices 表示"根据医生的医嘱；遵医嘱"。例：

Some kinds of powerful medications were given to her to the doctor's instructions. 遵医嘱，给她服用了一些强效药物。

4. And that really worked for relieving Mr. Li's pain and pressure. 这些治疗措施确实有助于缓解李先生的病痛和压力。

that... 指代前文所提到的情况，worked 表示"产生效果、有效、有助"。例：

That was a good decision as long as it worked for you. 只要对你有用，就是个明智的决定。

Section B

1. No headache or short-breath. Spirit, appetite and sleep is well. Normal urine and stool. 无头痛或气短。精神、食欲和睡眠良好。大小便正常。

2. Avoid getting fatigued and catching cold. 避免疲劳和着凉。

avoid sth. /doing sth. 表示"避免……/ 避免做……"。例：

He was always careful to avoid embarrassment. 他总是很小心地避免尴尬。

I avoid working in places which are too public. 我避免在过于抛头露面的地方工作。

3. Discharge medications: Benazepril tablets (10mg, po, qd); Pregabalin capsules (75mg, po, qn) 出院用药：洛丁新片（10mg，口服，每日）；普瑞巴林胶囊（75mg，口服，每夜）。

po. 口服；qd. 每日；qn. 每夜。例：

10mg, po, qd 每天白天口服 1 次，每次 10 毫克。

75mg, po, qn 每天晚上口服 1 次，每次 75 毫克。

4. Return to the hospital for examinations regularly and whenever uncomfortable. 请你定期回医院复查，有不适症状随时就诊。

whenever uncomfortable 在原句中为省略句，其完整形式应为 whenever you are

uncomfortable。例：

I recommend that you avoid processed foods whenever possible. 我建议你尽量不要食用加工好的食品。

Unit 9

Section A

1. It's too early to lose weight 现在减肥还太早。

too...to... 表示"太……而（不能）……"。例：

We were too slow to miss the bus. 我们动作太慢了以至于错过了公交车。

2. He is always being stressed for his job. 他总是因为工作而紧张万分。

be always/ constantly doing sth. 表示"总是……"。

与陈述性词组 always do sth. 不同，be always doing 常表达说话人的态度、情绪或评价。例：

She is always giving me a help hand whenever I am in trouble. 每当我有困难，她总是出手帮助。（表示出赞赏的评价。）

3. Remember, the chair is the killer. 记住，椅子就是个杀手。

本句意思是说久坐对健康不利，人们应当戒掉椅子，从"坐"姿中解放出来。

4. You'd better lose weight as fast as you can. 你最好尽快减肥。

as fast as you can 表示"尽你所能得快"；as...as... 表示"和……一样"。例：

This film is as interesting as that one. 这部电影和那部一样有趣。

Section B

1. The First Six Weeks after Caesarean Section 剖宫产手术后的首六周。

the first... (time) 指首段时间。例：

Free service is provided to all exhibitors for the first 3 hours. 大会在头三个小时提供免费服务。

2. A caesarean section is a surgical procedure in which a baby is born through a cut made in the mother's abdominal wall and uterus. 剖宫产手术是通过剖开母亲的腹壁及子宫而取出胎儿的外科手术。

A caesarean section is a surgical procedure 为主句，句意为"剖宫产手术是一个外科手术"。

in which 用于定语从句中，作关系副词。在本句中，in which 后的句子部分均为修饰 a surgical procedure 的定语从句。

3. Let her get as much rest as she can. 让她得到尽可能多的休息时间。

该句为祈使句（Imperative Sentence）。祈使句是用于表达命令、请求、劝告、警告、禁止等的句子。例：

Go and wash hands. 去洗手。（表示命令。）

Be quiet, please. 请安静。（表示请求。）

Look out! Danger! 小心！危险！（表示警告。）

No littering! 禁止乱扔垃圾！（表示禁止。）

4. ...her lower abdominal muscles and pelvic floor muscles will have weakened after pregnancy, and need strengthening.……在怀孕后，她的腹肌和盆底肌一定是有所削弱的，她需要锻炼这些肌肉。

5. ...to offer abdominal support, which can reduce pain and be worn for comfort for the first

six weeks.……以支撑腹部。（穿着）这些衣物是可以缓解疼痛的，并且在术后首六周（这样穿着）很舒适。

句中的 which 引导了一个非限制性定语从句。非限制性定语从句是对主句内容或先行词的补充、解释或附加说明。主句与从句之间一般用逗号分开。翻译时，常常可单独翻译。

6. The key of the nursing is that the mother must be kind to herself. 护理的关键是产妇一定要善待自己。

本句意思是说产妇一定要知道剖宫产后如何照顾自己，爱护自己是避免伤害和顺利康复的唯一方法。

Unit 10

Section A

1. Lily has Mr. Wang hold the ball in one hand, slowly raise the arm, fold the fingers and grasp the ball. 莉莉让王先生一手拿小球，慢慢抬高手臂，把手指合拢，抓握小球。

have sb. do.“让某人做某事”，后面跟由不带 to 的不定式构成的复合结构。例：

Don't forget to have him come. 别忘了让他来。

2. Mr. Wang was hospitalized with an intracerebral haemorrhage which led to the left limb dysfunction. 王先生突发脑出血入院，左侧肢体功能障碍。

which led to the left limb dysfunction 为定语从句，修饰先行词 an intracerebral haemorrhage; be hospitalized 表示“住院”。例：

He had a bad cold and was hospitalized for a month. 他患重感冒，住院一个月。

lead to 表示“引起，造成，导致”。例：

To much work and too little rest often leads to illness. 过多的工作、过少的休息常会引起疾病。

3. This makes the family members feel hopeful. 这让家属看到了希望。

make sb./sth. do 表示“使（做某事或成为）……”，跟由不带 to 的不定式构成的复合结构。例：

The light makes my eyes ache. 那光照得我眼睛疼。

4. Lily has kept giving her a daily massage and turn-over practice. 丽丽坚持给她按摩，做翻身练习。

keep doing sth. 表示“一直做某事，不断做某事”。例：

You shouldn't keep thinking about it. 你不应该老想它。

Section B

1. Many people with diseases such as spinal cord injury, stroke, and cerebral palsy will be at home for recuperation after surgery. 不少脊髓损伤、中风、脑瘫等患者术后都会回家休养。

such as 表示“例如”。例：

They export a lot of fruit, such as oranges, lemons, etc. 他们出口大量水果，如橘子、柠檬等。

2. But in most cases, some patients will be confined to bed forever. 可很多时候，患者一躺下就再也站不起来了。

be confined to 表示“被限制在（狭窄范围内）”。例：

He is confined to the house by illness for a week. 他因生病待在房子里一周了。

3. Successful rehabilitation can help these patients recover to an ideal health level or even help them regain their working ability. 成功的康复护理工作有助于患者恢复到理想的健康状态或重获工作能力。

help sb. (to) do sth. 表示“帮助某人做某事”。例：

Mr. Black helped me (to) solve it. 布莱克先生帮助我解决了此事。

听 力 原 文

Unit 1 Welcome to Nursing School

Section A My roommate Lily is in Nursing class 1.

Ⅱ. Listen and number the pictures1 to 4 in the order you hear them.

Mary is giving an injection.

Nancy is taking BP.

Nursing Class 1 is practicing nursing etiquette.

We are having a nursing practice class.

Ⅲ. Listen again and match the persons with what they are doing now.

Mary is giving an injection.

Nancy is taking BP.

Nursing class 1 is practicing nursing etiquette.

We are having a nursing practice class.

Unit 2 Go to Hospital

Section A What's the matter with Mary?

Ⅱ. Listen and number the pictures 1 to 4 in the order you hear them.

1. A: What's the matter with you?
   B: I have a fever.
   A: Let me take your temperature.
2. A: What's the matter with you?
   B: I have a sore throat.
   A: You should drink some hot tea with honey.
3. A: What's the matter with you?
   B: I have a toothache.
   A: You should see a dentist.
4. A: What's the matter with you?
   B: I cut myself.
   A: You should put some medicine and dress the wound.

Ⅲ. Listen again and match the symptoms with what advice they should take.

1. A: What's the matter with you?
   B: I have a fever.
   A: Let me take your temperature.
2. A: What's the matter with you?
   B: I have a sore throat.

A: You should drink some hot tea with honey.

3. A: What's the matter with you?
   B: I have a toothache.
   A: You should see a dentist.
4. A: What's the matter with you?
   B: I cut myself.
   A: You should put some medicine and dress the wound.

Unit 3 Treatment (Triage)

Section A Where is the registration office?

Ⅱ. Listen and number the pictures1 to 4 in the order you hear them.

1. Mr. Li is queuing for registration at the lobby on the first floor.
2. Ms. Chen is getting the medicine at the pharmacy at the corner.
3. My sister is waiting to see the doctor outside the Medical Department.
4. Doctor Zhang is examining the patient in the examination room on the second floor.

Ⅲ. Listen again and match the people with what and where they are doing.

1. A: Where is Mr. Li?
   B: He is queuing for registration at the lobby on the first floor.
2. A: Where is Ms. Chen?
   B: She is getting the medicine at the pharmacy at the corner.
3. A: Where is my sister?
   B: She is waiting to see the doctor outside the Medical Department.
4. A: Where is Doctor Zhang?
   B: He is examining the patient in the examination room on the second floor.

Unit 4 Giving Injections

Section A How terrible the injection is!

Ⅱ. Listen and number the pictures1 to 4 in the order you hear them.

The child is curious about being sterilized his skin.

Emily is careful to do a skin test.

The baby is calm when the nurse gives him IV fluids.

The boy is scared of being given an injection.

Ⅲ. Listen again and match emotions with the types of treatment.

The child is curious about being sterilized his skin.

Emily is careful to do a skin test.

The baby is calm when the nurse gives him IV fluids.

The boy is scared of being given an injection.

Unit 5 Drug Treatment

Section A The medicine is wonderful.

Ⅱ. Listen and number the pictures1 to 4 in the order you hear them.

Lily should rub the ointment when she needs.

Julia should read the instruction before taking the medicine.

Mary should take in oxygen once a day at bedtime.

Dina should take western medicine two tablets three times a day on an empty stomach.

Ⅲ. Listen again and match the medicine type with medication mode.

Lily should rub the ointment when she needs.

Julia should read the instruction before taking the medicine.

Mary should take in oxygen once a day at bedtime.

Dina should take western medicine two tablets three times a day on an empty stomach.

Unit 6 Medical Examination

Section A I would like to make an appointment.

Ⅱ. Listen and number the pictures1 to 4 in the order you hear them.

1. Health form filling—begins at 7:00 am.
2. Chest X-ray—begins at 9:00 am.
3. Lung's capacity measurement—begins at 8:30 am.
4. Talking about medical history to doctors—begins at 11:00 am.

Ⅲ. Listen again and match the items with when they begin.

1. Health form filling—begins at 7:00 am.
2. Chest X-ray—begins at 9:00 am.
3. Lung's capacity measurement—begins at 8:30 am.
4. Talking about medical history to doctors—begins at 11:00 am.

Unit 7 Admitted to Hospital

Section A How can I order a hospital bed?

Ⅱ. Listen and number the pictures 1 to 4 in the order you hear them.

1. Lily is writing the nursing notes.
2. John is transferring the patient to the Internal Medicine Department
3. Linda is checking the medical records.
4. Mary is reserving the hospital beds.

Ⅲ. Listen again and match the person with what they are doing now.

1. Lily is writing the nursing notes.
2. John is transferring the patient to the Internal Medicine Department
3. Linda is checking the medical records.
4. Mary is reserving the hospital beds.

Unit 8 Discharging from the Hospital

Section A My discharge summary is no see.

Ⅱ. Listen and number the pictures1 to 4 in the order you hear them.

Dr. Liu makes a ward-round from 9:00 to 10:00 in the morning.

Dr. Smith completes discharge summaries after the ward-round.

Head nurse gives medication instructions to the patients before the patients leave the hospital.

Student nurses tidy up the wards after the patients leave the hospital.

Ⅲ. Listen again and match the nursing invention with time.

Dr. Liu makes a ward-round from 9:00 to 10:00 in the morning.

Dr. Smith completes discharge summaries after the ward-round.

Head nurse gives medication instructions to the patients before the patients leave the hospital.

Student nurses tidy up the wards after the patients leave the hospital.

Unit 9 Health Education

Section A You should eat fluids.

Ⅱ. Listen and number the pictures1 to 4 in the order you hear them.

1. She must sleep in supine position to avoid choke.
2. She should eat fluids to be easy for absorption.
3. Your leg has to be in traction to help the recovery.
4. You'd better go for a massage to promote the blood circulation.

Ⅲ. Listen again and match the therapy method with health guidance.

1. She must sleep in supine position to avoid choke.
2. She should eat fluids to be easy for absorption.
3. Your leg has to be in traction to help the recovery.
4. You'd better go for a massage to promote the blood circulation.

Unit 10 Rehabilitation Instruction

Section A Nursing in the Rehabilitation Department

Ⅱ. Listen and number the pictures 1 to 4 in the order you hear them.

1. Bob's grandfather is giving acupuncture a whirl.
2. Mr. Mark is helping his wife with physical training.
3. Mary is having a high fever and her mother is helping Mary cool down with a cold towel.
4. Mr. Black suffered a stroke a month ago. Now he is practicing walking with a walker.

Ⅲ. Listen again and match the person with what they are doing now.

1. Bob's grandfather is giving acupuncture a whirl.
2. Mr. Mark is helping his wife with physical training.
3. Mary is having a high fever and her mother is helping Mary cool down with a cold towel.
4. Mr. Black suffered a stroke a month ago. Now he is practicing walking with a walker.

课 文 翻 译

Unit 1

Section A Reading

我的阿姨永葆青春

我的阿姨詹妮夫是一名护士长。她现在在澳大利亚。她就职于一所大型医院。

成为一名护士，是她的梦想。从高中毕业以后，她在护士学校就读三年，成为了一名护士生。在学校的三年时间里，她努力学习护理知识，勤奋练习护理技巧。在通过护士执业资格考试后，她毕业并且成为了一名注册护士。在这家医院，她已经工作了 20 多年。

虽然她已年逾四十，但是假如有人问到她的年龄，她总会这样回答："亲爱的，长大成人是一件很可怕的事。"

我为我的阿姨骄傲。

Section B

伟大的护士——南丁格尔

她本可以拥有轻松舒适的生活，但却选择了辛勤工作、照顾病患。弗洛伦斯·南丁格尔是世界上最伟大的护士之一。每年的 5 月 12 日，她生日的那一天，人们会共同庆祝"国际护士节"，以纪念她给予众人的博爱与帮助。

1820 年，南丁格尔出生于意大利佛罗伦萨的一个富裕家庭。24 岁的南丁格尔告诉父母，她想成为一名护士。但他们并不同意。因为这个家庭已经足够富裕，他们更愿意让女儿成为一名家庭主妇。在那时，护士这个职业并不能得到尊重。但南丁格尔坚持她的梦想。她去德国学习如何当一名护士。那时，没有护士学校，她只能通过实践来学习。

在 1854 年的战争中，南丁格尔和一支 38 人的护理队伍，从英格兰出发，前往土耳其附近护理受伤的士兵。是她让战地医院的卫生环境得到改善。

在晚上，她需要照顾伤者。提着灯的她，被士兵们称为"提灯女神"。

在战后的 1860 年，南丁格尔开办了世界上第一所护士学校。同时，她还在不断为医院改善而努力，并致力于完善和规范护士职责。1910 年，她在英格兰伦敦逝世，享年 90 岁。

1912 年，南丁格尔的生日被定为"国际护士节"。

Unit 2

Section A Reading

雪莉·布莱恩医生忙了一下午

今天下午，我和我的朋友们去了学校诊所。雪莉·布莱恩医生在这家学校诊所里工作。

第一个去诊所的是玛丽。她是护理 4 班的学生。这一天很冷，但她只穿了一条很短的裙子。她面色苍白，一直咳嗽。她告诉医生她感到头疼。仔细检查后，雪莉医生告诉她，她感冒了，并不严重。雪莉医生建议她每天服药三次，坚持三天。在寒冷的天气里要记得穿暖和的衣服。

我的室友萨拉是第二个去学校诊所的。她说她肚子痛。雪莉医生问她午饭吃了什么。萨拉说她吃了四个大汉堡，一大杯加冰的可口可乐，外加一大盒冰激凌。雪莉医生说："这顿午餐真是太过丰盛了！嗯，没什么大碍。记住多运动，少吃点！"

我是最后一个去学校诊所的。我叫莉莉。我来诊所是因为我从自行车上摔了下来，伤到了右脚。雪莉医生让我躺下，把一些冰放在我的右脚上。过了一会儿，我感觉好多了。雪莉医生告诉我，回家后的头两天里，需要用冰在右脚上每小时冷敷 5 分钟。"卧床休息一周，"雪丽医生说。

多么忙碌的一下午啊！

Section B

医院

医院是给病人或者需要看医生的人提供治疗和护理的地方，如孕妇。医院也可能是一个医学研究中心或者是一所培训医生、护士和其他医疗工作者的学校。

医院可以分为综合性医院和专科医院。综合性医院有很多不同的科室，如内科、外科、儿科、妇产科、牙科、中医科。不同年龄段的病人和不同伤病的患者都可以在综合性医院进行治疗。其他的医院提供更专门的治疗。比如有些医院为慢性病患者提供治疗和长期治疗的设施。另外一些医院或者只接收某个年龄段的病人，如儿童，或者只接收某种特殊疾病的患者，如结核病人。

医院由两个主要部门构成：门诊部和住院部，此外还有急诊室。门诊部设有很多诊室。住院部有许多病房和重症监护室。病房可以分为很多种，如内科病房、外科病房、产科病房、隔离病房、观察病房。每个病房都有几张病床。

医院的工作人员由医生、护士和其他医务人员组成。根据专业的不同，医生可分为内科医生、外科医生、眼科医生、耳鼻喉科医生、牙医等。医生和护士都照顾病人。对于医生，首先强调的是医学知识，而对于护士，首先强调的是康复技术。人们说：医生治疗疾病；护士治疗病人。医院的病人每天只能看几分钟的医生。但是他们见护士的频率反而很高，因为护士为医院的患者提供了主要的护理与康复服务。他们对患者进行全天 24 小时的看护。

Unit 3

Section A　Reading

多么尴尬的一次经历啊

我叫山姆，是一个来自美国的生意人。去年暑假因为工作需要到英国出差五天，可能是因为太累了，而且有点感冒了，到了伦敦的第二天就发起了高烧，为了不影响接下来的工作，我立即到当地一家综合性医院看病。

到了医院之后，分诊护士告知我应该挂内科，并且告诉了我内科在三楼的尽头。于是我马上乘坐电梯到达了三楼，径直走到了尽头，由于有点头痛，我并没有看清楚科室牌就排起队来。可是过了一会儿我觉得有点不对劲，怎么排队的全部都是女的呢？我抬头一看科室牌，天啊，这里是妇科。正当我不知所措的时候，妇科医生对我说：小伙子，内科在上面一层楼，正好在这间房间的正上方。我忍不住问了一句，这里不是三楼吗？这时周围的人都笑了起来，其中有人对我说了一句：你肯定不是英国人。

多么尴尬的一次经历啊！

Section B Extensive Reading

圣诞节急诊

十二月二十五日，急诊室里异乎寻常地安静。我是当天的分诊护士。我想不会有什么病人来的。当我正叹息着圣诞节还要工作的时候，五个人出现在我的办公桌前：一个面色苍白的妇女和四个小孩儿。

我问道："你们都病了吗？"

"嗯。"她虚弱地回答道，低下了头。

但是当他们开始描述现在的病情时，事情就有点让人不确定了。其中两个孩子头痛，但是他们的头痛并没有伴随着通常出现的肢体症状，像抱头或者试着让头保持不动等。还有，两个孩子说耳朵痛，但只有一个能告诉我是哪只耳朵痛。孩子的母亲诉说她有咳嗽症状，但咳嗽好像是用力装出来的。

事情有点不对头，但是我也没说什么，只是解释说，过一阵儿医生才会来给她检查。她回答说："不着急，医院里挺暖和的。"接诊员填好这个家庭的登记表后，出于直觉，我查看了一下。上面没写地址——他们无家可归。候诊室里很暖和。

我回到护士室，讲述了候诊室里这无家可归的一家子的事。原本抱怨圣诞节还要上班的护士们都转而对在圣诞节只祈求温暖的这家人感到非常同情。这个团队马上展开行动，就好像我们对待医疗紧急情况一样，只不过这次是"圣诞节急诊"。

圣诞节这天，医院食堂免费给我们提供一顿饭，于是我们都把饭领回来，为我们的圣诞客人准备了一次宴会。还需要一些礼物，我们从不同的部门收集了糖果、水果和其他可以提供的东西。我们的团队工作严肃，就像满足当天其他患者的需要一样，我们尽力满足这家人只想过一个温暖圣诞节的愿望。

后来，当这家人走到门前要离开的时候，那个四岁的孩子跑回来，给了我一个拥抱，并在我的耳边悄悄地说："谢谢你，今天你是我们家的天使。"

Unit 4

Section A Reading

我给病人打针的经历

我已经在医院做了一个月实习护士。护士长今天上午让我给病人打针。在学校时我给同学打过针，但这次不同——为真正的病人服务！我有点既兴奋又紧张。我生病时，打过几次针，其中有些让我感觉到打针的疼。我想知道当我把针头刺入皮肤时，我会不会导致病人疼痛。打针是我的职责，它也有利于病人，所以我必须按我的职责去做。

首先我回忆了我将遵守的五个准确：给予准确的患者、准确的药物、按准确的剂量、用准确的途径和在准确的时间。然后我检查了药物，确保一切都准备好了。我要表现出我是胜任的。仔细地清洁双手后，我见到了我的病人，她需要注射盘尼西林。我询问她是否对此药物过敏，接着给她做了皮试。20分钟后，结果显示她不过敏。在消毒皮肤后，我快速、仔细地把针头插入。病人很配合。我成功了！

Section B

静脉输液——了解一些事情

静脉输液是如今医院最重要的治疗手段之一。医务工作者和病人都应该谨慎使用静脉输液。

介绍

Ⅳ的意思是“在静脉内”。静脉输液通常称为点滴。静脉途径是能最快遍及全身的给液和给药途径。

用法

静脉输液给药通常适用于不能口服治疗或者注射治疗的病人。它可以用于输液（如纠正脱水）、纠正电解质紊乱、给药和输血。

部位

静脉输液最常见部位是手部。当手部静脉不合适时，可以通过胳膊处静脉进行点滴。

速度

大部分情况下，病人在固定时间内接受药物治疗直到输液袋输完。液体不能滴太快，必须慢点滴，以免病人负荷不了。

副作用

虽然一般来讲静脉用药是安全的，它也会导致轻度或危险的副作用。静脉用药很快作用于人体，所以副作用，如疼痛、感染、血块、过敏反应和其他效果会很快显现出来。大部分情况下，一名医疗服务提供者会对你的输液全程进行观察，有时候也会在之后的一段时间（进行观察）。

静脉用药是把药物送入人体血流的快速且有效的方式，但是任何事物都有两面性，所以不要对其滥用。如果有任何不适，马上联系医生或护士。

Unit 5

Section A Reading

神奇之药

一个人正在集市上卖药。开始的时候他卖的只是一美元一瓶的感冒药。

许多人都想买这个感冒药，那个人的助手收钱然后把感冒药分发给人们。

然后，当有一大群人的时候，那个人举起一个非常小的瓶子，大声说道：“先生们，女士们，这就是你们一直等着要的药——治疗衰老的药。只要喝一瓶这种药，你就可以永生。”

“先生们，女士们，”那个人继续说道，“这个神奇药，我不打算收你们100美元一瓶，不会的，我只收你们10美元一瓶。我的朋友们，好好想想，只要10美元你就可以永生。”

人群中的大部分人不相信他所说的话。

有个人大声说道：“如果这个药可以让你永生，为什么你自己不喝呢？”

另外一个人大声喊道：“是啊，你看起来至少有60岁了。”

“谢谢你，先生，谢谢你，”那个人回答道，“我很高兴你那么说。我真正的年龄是329岁。”

人们对他说的话嗤之以鼻，但是仍有几个人想相信那个人。在他的助手经过的时候，其中的一个人问他的助手：“是真的吗？”“他有329岁？”

“不要问我，”那个助手说，“我才仅仅为他工作了150年。”

Section B

新型抗癌药

科学家们研制出一种新的抗癌药物。到目前为止，他们只在实验室动物身上进行了测试。这种药物的目的是进入和杀死癌细胞，而不是健康细胞。

首先，药物进入癌细胞并停止其血液供应。然后它释放毒素来破坏癌细胞。

剑桥大写的研究人员进行了这项研究。一份学校报告称这种药物为“抗癌智能炸弹”。拉姆是研究人员之一。他说他的团队必须解决三个问题。他们必须找到一种方法来摧毁血管，然后阻止新生血管的生长。但是他们也需要血管供给化学物质来消灭癌症。

因此，研究人员设计了一个由两部分组成的“纳米细胞”。这个细胞是用纳米或者十亿分之一米来测量的。

科学家们说，它足够小，可以通过癌症的血管，但它太大，无法进入正常血管。纳米细胞的表面也有助于它们避免自然防御。

科学家们把这个细胞设计成气球内的气球。他们用一种使血管死亡的药物填满了外面的部分。这样会切断血液供应，将纳米细胞置于癌细胞内。然后，纳米细胞缓慢释放药物杀死癌细胞。

研究小组说，这种治疗方法比其他治疗方法更好地杀死癌细胞和避免健康细胞。未经治疗的患了癌症的小鼠存活二十天。科学家说，用目前最好的治疗方法治疗这个小鼠，小鼠存活三十天。在这项研究中，他们说用纳米细胞治疗的老鼠中有百分之八十的寿命超过六十五天。

科学家们说，在新药能够在人类身上进行试验之前，还需要进行更多的研究。

Unit 6

Section A Reading

体格检查的重要性

体格检查用于检查你身体的总体健康情况。它能检查身体的很多器官和其他部位，例如心脏、肺部、视力、胃等。年度体格检查是十分重要的，它可以防止染上重大疾病而不自知，保证你和你家人的健康长寿。

年度体格检查对于你和你的家庭来说都非常重要，它能够预防严重的疾病，保障健康长寿。父母通常都会确保孩子接受年度体格检查，然而年检在成人年中也越来越重要。它通常包括常规检查、心脏检查、肺部检查等。

为了节省时间，去体检之前预约是十分必要的。在日常生活中，电话预约和网上预约都非常流行。你必须提前 24 小时打电话预约或在网上进行登记预约。当预约时，你需要提供姓名、性别、联系电话等个人信息。并且，你最好事先知道分别在哪里做何种检查。

在体检过程中，请诚实面对医生，确保你毫无保留地说出关于你健康的问题或担心，即便是很小的一点也不例外。体检后，仔细倾听医生的建议，大胆提出疑问。

有两种简单的方法能够延年益寿

加拿大关于访客和工作者的体检要求：坚持年度体格检查和养成良好的生活习惯。我们任何可能产生疾病的情况下都要采取措施防止疾病。每天运动、保持健康的体重和不吸烟，这些重要的方面是必不可少的。

Section B

如果你打算去加拿大的时间在六个月以内，你不需要体检。如果在六个月以上，你就需要去体检了。还有其他一些情况，你也必须体检：你已经连续居住六个月或以上，或者你在当地参加具有需重点维护公共安全的工作，又或者你要申请父母及祖父母的超级签证。

下面几种情况的工作需要进行体格检查：

1. 往年中，访问或居住满六个月及以上的农业工人；

2. 与人群接触密切的想过工作，如：健康科学领域的工作人员，检验人员；
3. 被加拿大高校录取的医学生，小学、中学教师或与儿童工作相关的教师；
4. 居家式照顾小孩、老人和残疾人的工作者；
5. 日间托儿所的工作者；等等。

然而，并不是所有的医生都能进行体检，你必须找到名单上专门的体检机构，他们会给你做完整的体格检查。体检结束后，体检医生会给你体检结果。如果检查有任何问题，签证办公室会以书面形式联系你。如果你想要一份体检报告，请在当场告诉医生。

谈及费用，你必须在当场付清所有费用。如果政府未通过你的申请，将不退还体检费。

Unit 7

Section A Reading

我住院了！

生病或不舒服的时候，我会去医院，到门诊部做一下常规检查。三天前，我感到非常难受，于是去了医院。挂号以后，我向医生主诉了自己的症状，已经呕吐三天了。医生给我进行了体检，并让我做了一些医学检验，其中包括血液检测、大便检查以及尿液检查。他告诉我，我的病情有些严重，必须住院接受进一步诊断或治疗。我听从医生的建议，并从他那儿拿到了入院通知。

我需要办理入院手续。首先，我向护士出示了医生给我开的入院通知，然后我就去了付款大厅支付了预付定金。

填写完入院登记表，并支付了预付定金后，一位友善的护士带我去了我的病房。这位护士对我说道："这儿就是你的病房了；你的病床号是310A。这个是呼叫灯。只要按下按钮，护士就会立刻来提供帮助和护理了。"她还提醒我医院的探视时间是早上八点到八点半，下午两点半到三点。

过了一会儿，病房护士进来问我是否对任何药物过敏，比如说青霉素。事实上，我也不知道。于是这位病房护士为我做了皮试。她还提醒我如果我感到发痒或是呼吸困难，一定立刻告诉她。

从我踏进医院的那一刻起，我的家人和我就盼望着出院的那一天。由于我自己非常积极地配合治疗，我的症状和病情得到了控制。

Section B

入院

病人的入院是进入医院的正规程序。当病人住进医院时，了解住院程序是非常重要的。病房的环境、护理体系都将介绍给住院患者。这一过程也是为评估病人临床状况和护理需要而收集资料的一种方法。

对于患者来说，他们办理入院手续时，需要检查入院卡、入院申请表、身份证、国家医疗保险IC卡及相关证书（证明患有主要疾病或严重受伤的卡片等）以及以前的医疗记录。入院卡是由患者的主治医生提供的。入院申请表包括个人资料、病史、入院原因和将采取的治疗等。病人或其家属必须在入院前填写入院表格，并在上面签字。病人的病史是医生或其他医护人员通过询问特定问题获得的信息；病史中包含患者本人提供的信息或者其他了解患者的任何人所提供的病情信息，通过提供有用的信息帮助患者形成诊断并提供合理的医疗服务。

对于护士来说，当被通知病人要到来的时候，护士们应该把病房准备好。由护士通知患者入院的信息以及数据，在通知的时间内办理好所有的住院手续，否则将不予保留床位。不能让病人自己单独去病房，因为他可能会迷路，会跌倒，或者受到伤害。病人一入院，护士就应该给他做体检。这样做是因为医院需要一个病人状况的完整记录。

Unit 8

Section A Reading

李先生的住院期

一周前，李先生因为严重的头晕、视线模糊及胸痛被收治入院。

根据主诉，李先生有很长的高血压病史。他的主治医生卢医生决定为他做一次全面检查。

入院前三天，李先生都忙于应付各种检查项目。不久之后，为李先生所做的一系列必要的入院检查就已经全部完成。这些检查包括血、尿常规、大便常规、凝血常规、胸片及心电图，检查结果均显示正常。检查中使用了多普勒彩超。彩超结果显示李先生有脂肪肝和动脉硬化。

根据所有的检查结果分析，卢医生为李先生进行了细致的诊断。根据医嘱，李先生住院期间接受了一系列必要的治疗。针对改善血液循环、控制血压及改善情绪和睡眠等方面的措施被用于对他的治疗。这些治疗措施确实有助于缓解其病痛与压力。

经过精心的诊治和护理，李先生的情绪和睡眠有所改善，其头晕、视线模糊及胸痛等症状有所缓解，其本人也慢慢变得乐观开朗起来。

Section B Extensive Reading

<table>
<tr><th colspan="6">出院医嘱</th></tr>
<tr><td>姓名</td><td>李源</td><td>年龄</td><td>68</td><td>性别</td><td>男</td></tr>
<tr><td>所属科室</td><td>神经内科</td><td>病床号</td><td>5</td><td>住院号</td><td>1407151</td></tr>
<tr><td>出院日期</td><td>2014 年 6 月 20 日</td><td colspan="2">出院情况</td><td colspan="2">无头痛或气短。精神、食欲和睡眠良好。大小便正常</td></tr>
<tr><td colspan="6">注意事项</td></tr>
<tr><td colspan="6">1. 充分休息、适量运动；
2. 避免疲劳和着凉；
3. 严格监控日常饮食中钠和脂肪的摄入量</td></tr>
<tr><td colspan="6">出院用药</td></tr>
<tr><td colspan="6">1. 洛丁新片，每天白天口服 1 次，每次 10 毫克；
2. 普瑞巴林胶囊，每天晚上口服 1 次，每次 75 毫克；
3. 阿普唑仑片，每天晚上口服 1 次，每次 0.4 毫克</td></tr>
<tr><td colspan="6">出院指导</td></tr>
<tr><td colspan="6">1. 监测血压值和血脂值；
2. 定期使用多普勒彩超进行肝脏和动脉常规复查；
3. 定期回医院复查，有不适症状随时就诊</td></tr>
<tr><td colspan="6">医生签名：卢笛</td></tr>
</table>

Unit 9

Section A Reading

减肥还太早

比尔是一个画家。他是个体型肥胖的男人。他的工作总是很紧张。

一天，比尔觉得身体不舒服，于是他来到了医院。医生对他进行诊断后发现，比尔就要因肥胖而致病了。

医生建议他："先生，你该试着减减肥了。肥胖是导致高血压的一个重要原因。高血压将会危害你的健康。"

"医生，我该怎么办呢？" 比尔沮丧地问。

医生告诉比尔："记住，椅子就是个杀手。不要长时间坐着。你应该多做运动，并且不能熬夜。你最好能尽快减肥。注意自己的血压。"

比尔很勉强地笑了笑说："恐怕要我减肥已经太迟了。我总是坐在椅子上，对着一副画一画就是几小时。"

医生试着鼓励他："减肥永远都不会太晚的！你能做到的！"

"医生你是认真的吗？减肥永远都不晚？" 比尔问道。

"是的。先生，你可以高兴点了。" 医生回答道。

"永远都不晚，所以对我来说减肥应该还太早呢！谢谢你，医生！" 比尔开心地说着并离开了医院。

Section B

剖宫产手术后的首六周

剖宫产手术是通过剖开母亲的腹壁及子宫，取出胎儿的外科手术。剖宫产手术后，产妇通常会留院 3~5 天。术后第一周，产妇就能回到家中。以下是剖宫产术后首六周的护理提示：

让她得到尽可能多的休息时间。

不允许她拿起任何比一个婴儿更重的物品。当她拿起物品时，注意她的后背（是否感到不适）。

鼓励她每天散步。这对她的身心健康都有好处。

帮助她完成一些盆底运动。必须要告诉她：在怀孕后，她的腹肌和盆底肌一定是有所削弱的，她需要锻炼这些肌肉。

让她多吃健康的高纤维食物，并且要大量饮水。每日如此，以避免便秘。

保持伤口的清洁和干燥。关注伤口是否有感染的症状（如伤口变红、疼痛、伤口肿大或是有异味排出）。

她必须要知道，穿着宽松的衣服是可以的。而有的人更喜欢穿高腰的紧身内衣，或是控制型内衣，以此支撑起腹部。（穿着）这些衣物是可以缓解疼痛的，并且，在术后首六周（这样穿着）很舒适。

对所有女人而言，照顾新生儿是一件很辛苦的事情，但更辛苦的是她们需要从剖宫产手术中恢复过来。护理的关键就是产妇一定要善待自己。

Unit 10

Section A Reading

康复护士的梦想

莉莉 5 年前从护理学校毕业，现在是康复中心的一名护士。她每天给病人打针、换药、按摩、帮助病人做康复训练。

莉莉现在正在病房，帮助王先生用小球进行手部功能康复训练。莉莉让王先生一手拿小球，慢慢抬高手臂，把手指合拢，抓握小球。20 多天前，王先生突发脑出血入院，左侧肢体功能障碍。经过这些天的练习，王先生现在已经可以抓住小球而不会掉落。这让家属看到了希望。

60 多岁的刘奶奶患了脑梗，在医院接受治疗。她刚入院时几乎动弹不得。一个多月以来，莉莉每天坚持给她按摩、翻身练习。现在，她已经能扶墙慢慢走路了。

这样的例子还有很多。看到这些病人渐渐康复，莉莉觉得自己的努力是值得的。哪怕工作再累，她也会坚守自己的岗位，能让更多的患者重新开始健康、快乐的生活，是她最大的愿望。

Section B Extensive Reading

你了解康复吗?

很多人对康复医学不太了解。不少脊髓损伤、中风、脑瘫等患者术后都会回家休养。大部分家属认为，病人能快速康复起来。可很多时候，患者一躺下就再也站不起来了。

成功的康复护理工作有助于患者恢复到理想的健康状态或重获工作能力。很遗憾，一些家属未能为患者的快速康复提供良好的家庭护理，患者因未能得到家人的康复护理而导致健康状况恶化。事实证明，一半以上的中风病人经过一年左右的康复治疗，基本能够实现日常生活的自理，而需要全部帮助的患者仅有 5% 。

语　法

Nouns（名词）

一、名词的概念和分类

表示人、事物或抽象概念的词叫做名词，可以分为专有名词和普通名词两大类（表 1)。专有名词是表示具体的人、事物、地点或机构的名称。普通名词是表示某类人或某类事物的名称，又可分为表示单个的人或事物的个体名词、表示一群人或一些事物的总称的集体名词、表示无法分为个体的物质名词、表示抽象概念的抽象名词四类。

此外，根据名词是否有复数形式，还可以把名词分为可数名词和不可数名词两大类。

表 1　名词的分类

专有名词			Einstein 爱因斯坦　Beijing 北京　CCTV 中国中央电视台
普通名词	可数名词	个体名词	book 书　kid 孩子　friend 朋友
		集体名词	family 家庭　class 班级　team 队
	不可数名词	物质名词	water 水　air 空气　bread 面包
		抽象名词	love 热爱　Chinese 汉语　success 成功

二、可数名词的复数形式

可数名词复数形式的构成规则如下：

1. 绝大多数名词的复数形式是在名词后加 -s。如：desk-desks，map-maps，book-books。

2. 以 /s/、/z/ 结尾和以辅音字母加 -o 结尾的名词构成复数形式时，要在其后加 -es，如：bus-buses，box-boxes。

3. 以字母 -f 或 -fe 结尾的名词构成复数形式时，要把 -f 或 -fe 改为 -v，再加 -es。如：life-lives，leaf-leaves。

4. 以辅音字母加 -y 结尾的名词构成复数形式时，要把 -y 改为 -i，再加 -es。如：baby-babies，country-countries。

5. 有些名词的复数形式变化不规则，需要单独记忆。常见的有：man-men，foot-feet，mouse-mice。

Pronouns（代词）

代词是指代人和事物的词，主要替代名词以及起名词作用的短语、不定式、动名词、从句或句子，以避免重复。代词分为八类，即人称代词、物主代词、反身代词、指示代词、疑问代词、不定代词、连接代词和关系代词。这里只介绍前六类。

一、人称代词

表示“我”“你”“他”“我们”“你们”“他们”的词称为人称代词。人称代词分为主格和宾格，其变化形式如表2：

表2 人称代词的数和格

数、格 / 人称	单数		复数	
	主格	宾格	主格	宾格
第一人称	I	me	we	us
第二人称	you	you	you	you
第三人称	he	him	they	them
	she	her		
	it	it		

二、物主代词

表示所有关系的代词称为物主代词。物主代词有形容词性物主代词和名词性物主代词两种，形式如表3：

表3 物主代词的分类

词义 / 词类	我的	你的	他的	她的	它的	我们的	你们的	他们的
形容词性	my	your	his	her	its	our	your	their
名词性	mine	yours	his	hers	its	ours	yours	theirs

三、反身代词

表示“我自己”“你自己”“他自己”“我们自己”“你们自己”“他们自己”的代词称为反身代词，其形式如表4：

表4 反身代词的数和人称

人称 / 数	第一人称	第二人称	第三人称
单数	myself	yourself	himself, herself, itself
复数	ourselves	yourselves	themselves

四、指示代词

表示“这个”“那个”“这些”“那些”等意思的代词称为指示代词。指示代词有this, that, these, those等，其指代关系如表5：

表5 指示代词的使用

指示代词	近指	远指	单数	复数
this	√		√	
that		√	√	
these	√			√
those		√		√

五、不定代词

不定代词表示没有指明的人或事。不定代词有：some（某个，某些），any（任何一个），no（没有），none（没有人，没有什么东西），many（许多），much（许多），few（少），little（少），each（各个），every（每个），one（一个，任何人），all（所有的，一切），both（两者都），either（二者之一），neither（二者都不），other（别的，其他），another（另一个）等。复合不定代词有：nobody（没有人），somebody（某人），anybody（任何人），nothing（没有东西），something（某事，某物），anything（任何事物）等。常用不定代词的用法区分如下：

1. all 和 both

all 表示两个以上的人或事物，**both** 表示“两者都……”。试比较以下两组句子：

All are here.
Both of them like the music.

She has read all the books about Harry Porter.
These two books are very interesting. I want both.

2. some 和 any

some 和 **any** 既可以修饰可数名词，也可以修饰不可数名词，但 any 常用在疑问句和否定句中，而 some 常用在肯定句中。试比较以下两组句子：

I have some pens.
Have you any pens?

Some sit, some stand.
Does any of you know Alice?

3. many 和 much

many 用来修饰或替代可数名词，**much** 用来修饰或替代不可数名词。试比较以下两组句子：

Many students were in the classroom this afternoon.
Much has been done to improve the work.

How many sisters do you have?
There is not much water left in the cup.

六、疑问代词

疑问代词包括 who, whom, whose, which 和 what 五个词。

Numerals（数词）

表示数目多少或顺序先后的词叫数词。数词分成两大类：基数词和序数词。表示“多少”的词叫基数词，如 one, hundred 等；表示“第几”的词叫序数词，如 first, hundredth。

一、基数词

最基本的基数词如下，其他的数词都可以由这些词组成。

one	(1)	twelve	(12)	forty	(40)
two	(2)	thirteen	(13)	fifty	(50)
three	(3)	fourteen	(14)	sixty	(60)
four	(4)	fifteen	(15)	seventy	(70)
five	(5)	sixteen	(16)	eighty	(80)
six	(6)	seventeen	(17)	ninety	(90)
seven	(7)	eighteen	(18)	a hundred	(100)
eight	(8)	nineteen	(19)	a thousand	(1,000)
nine	(9)	twenty	(20)	a million	(1,000,000)
ten	(10)	twenty-one	(21)	a billion	(1,000,000,000)
eleven	(11)	thirty	(30)		

二、序数词

序数词一般由基数词加 -th 构成，如 fourth, sixth, eleventh 等。以 -y 结尾的基数词构成序数词时，先把 -y 变为 -i，再加 -eth，如 twentieth, fortieth, fiftieth 等。还有一些词的构成变化不规则，如：

第一 first　　第二 second　　第三 third　　第五 fifth
第八 eighth　　第九 ninth　　第十二 twelfth

在日常生活中，序数词常被简化，一般规律是：阿拉伯数字后加相应序数词的末尾两个字母，如 1st, 2nd, 3rd, 4th, 21st, 30th, 105th。

数词用法的规则如下：

1. 编号的事物可用序数词或基数词加名词表示。例如：

the Fourth Lesson—Lesson Four

2. 有些编号的事物常用基数词表示。例如：

Room801, Bus No.1, Page56, the No.3 Middle School

3. 表示“年、月、日”时，“年”用基数词。例如：

June 5th, 1996；May1^{st}, 2017

4. 表示“几点钟”时使用基数词。例如：

four (o'clock), five past three, twenty to nine

Adjectives & Adverbs（形容词和副词）

一、形容词

用来修饰名词的词语都可以算作形容词。形容词一般在句子里充当表语、定语或补语，有时与其他词一起构成短语后作状语用。请看下面五个例句：

(1) We had a good time yesterday.

(2) The climate here is wet.

(3) The classroom is kept tidy.

(4) I was lying in bed, wide awake.

(5) We should respect the old and love the young.

例句 (1) 里的形容词作定语；句 (2) 里的形容词作表语；句 (3) 中的形容词作补语；句 (4) 中的形容词作状语；句 (5) 中的形容词由 the 修饰，相当于名词。

二、副　词

副词可以修饰动词、形容词、名词、其他副词或全句。副词的种类很多，常见的有时间副词、地点副词、方式副词、程度副词、频度副词、肯定（否定）副词、疑问副词、关系副词和连接副词等。请看下列例句：

(6) Bob often goes to school by bicycle.

(7) In 1928 Mickey Mouse first appeared in a cartoon film.

(8) Can you tell me how you did it?

(9) When do you go to school every day?

例句 (6) 里的 often 是频度副词；句 (7) 里的 first 是时间副词；句 (8) 里的 how 是连接副词；句 (9) 里的 when 是疑问副词。

三、形容词和副词的比较级与最高级

形容词和副词的比较等级分为原级、比较级和最高级。它们的变化形式分规则和不规则两种。规则变化有如下规律：

1．在单音节形容词后、少数以 -er，-ow，-ble，-ple 结尾的双音节形容词和少数副词后加 -er，-est 或 -r，-st。例如：

strong—stronger—strongest

clever—cleverer—cleverest

2．在以 -e 结尾的单音节形容词和少数副词后加 -r，-st。例如：

brave—braver—bravest

wide—wider—widest

3．形容词以一个辅音字母结尾，其前面的元音字母发短元音时，该辅音字母要双写，然后加 -er，-est，例如：

big—bigger—biggest

hot—hotter—hottest

4．辅音字母后加 -y 结尾的单音节及双音节形容词和少数副词（由形容词后缀 -ly 构成的副词除外）要将 -y 变为 -i，再加 -er, -est。例如：

easy—easier—easiest

early—earlier—earliest

5．在双音节和多音节形容词和大多数副词前可以加 more 和 most 分别构成比较级和最高级。例如：

important—more important—most important

quickly—more quickly—most quickly

6．常见形容词和副词的不规则变化如表6所列，需要熟记：

表6 常见形容词和副词的不规则变化表

原形	比较级	最高级
good	better	best
well	better	best
many	more	most
much	more	most
bad	worse	worst
badly	worse	worst
ill	worse	worst
little	less	least
far	farther	farthest
	further	furthest

Prepositions（介词）

介词是一种用来表示词与词、词与句之间的关系的虚词，在句中不能单独作句子成分。介词后面一般有名词、代词或相当于名词的其他词类、短语或从句作它的宾语。介词和它的宾语构成介词词组，在句中作状语、表语、补语或介词宾语。介词可以分为时间介词、地点介词、方式介词、原因介词和其他介词。

一、表示地点位置的介词

1．at，in，on，to，for

at（1）表示在小地方；（2）表示“在……附近，旁边”。

in（1）表示在大地方；（2）表示“在……范围之内”。

on 强调毗邻，接壤，表示“在……上面”。

to 表示“在……范围外”，不强调是否接壤；或表示“到……”。

2．above，over，on“在……上”

above 指“在……上方”，不强调是否垂直，与 **below** 相对；

over 指“垂直的上方”，与 **under** 相对，但 over 与物体有一定的空间，不直接接触。

on 表示“某物体上面”并与之接触。如：

（1）The bird is flying above my head.

（2）There is a bridge over the river.

（3）He put his watch on the desk.

3．below，under“在……下面”

under 表示“在……正下方”。

below 表示“在……下”，不一定在正下方。如：

There is a cat under the table. 桌子下面有只猫。

Please write your name below the line.　请在线下写您的姓名。

4．in front of，in the front of“在……前面”

in front of... 意思是“在……前面”，指甲物在乙物之前，两者互不包含；其反义词是 behind（在……的后面）。如：

There are some flowers in front of the house. 房子前面有些花卉。

in the front of 意思是“在……的前部”，即甲物在乙物的内部。反义词是 at the back of（在……范围内的后部）。如：

There is a blackboard in the front of our classroom. 我们的教室前边有一块黑板。

Our teacher stands in the front of the classroom. 我们的老师站在教室的前面。

5. beside，behind

beside 表示“在……旁边”；**behind** 表示“在……后面”。

二、表示时间的介词

1. in，on，at“在……时”

in 表示较长时间，如世纪、朝代、时代、年、季节、月及一般（非特指）的早、中、晚等。

如 in the 20th century，in the 1950s，in 1989，in summer，in January，in the morning，in one's life，in one's thirties 等。

on 表示具体某一天及其早、中、晚。

如 on May 1st，on Monday，on New Year's Day，on a cold night in January，on a fine morning，on Sunday afternoon 等。

at 表示某一时刻或较短暂的时间，或泛指圣诞节、复活节等。

如 at 3:20，at this time of year，at the beginning of，at the end of...，at the age of...，at Christmas，at night，at noon，at this moment 等。

[注意] 在 last，next，this，that，some，every 等词之前一律不用介词。如：We meet every day.

2. in，after“在……之后”

“in+ 段时间”表示将来的一段时间以后；

“after+ 段时间”表示过去的一段时间以后；

“after+ 将来的时间点”表示将来的某一时刻以后。

3. from，since“自从……”

from 仅说明什么时候开始，不说明某动作或情况持续多久；

since 表示“自（某具体时间）以来”，即该动作或情况一直持续到说话时，通常与完成时连用。如：

They have been close friends since childhood. 他们是从小玩到大的好朋友。

注意：

（1）since the war 是指“自从战争结束以来”。若表示“自从战争开始以来”，须说 since the beginning of the war。

（2）不要将 since 与 after 混淆。如：

He has worked here since 1965.
自从 1965 年以来，他一直在这儿工作。（指一段时间，强调时间段。）
He began to work here after 1965.
从 1965 年以后，他就开始在这儿工作。（指一点时间，强调时间点。）

4．after，behind“在……之后”

after 主要用于表示时间；**behind** 主要用于表示位置。

三、表示运动方向的介词

across，through“通过，穿过”

across“横过”，即从物体表面通过。

through“穿过”，即从物体内部穿过。

四、表示“在……之间”的介词

表示“在……之间”的介词在英语中属于方位介词，如 between，among。

between 指在两个人或两个事物之间；

among 指在三个或三个以上的人或事物之间。

五、表示其他意义的介词

1．on，about“关于”

on 表示书、文章或演说是严肃的或学术性的，可供专门研究这一问题的人阅读；

about 表示内容较为普通，不那么正式。

2．by，with，in 表示“方法、手段、工具”

by“以……方法、手段”或泛指某种交通工具；

with 表示“用……工具、手段”，一般接具体的工具和手段；

in 表示“用……方式，用……语言（语调、笔墨、颜色）等”。

3．except，besides“除了”

except 除……之外，不包括在内；

besides 除……之外，包括在内。如：

Except for Mr. Wang，we went to see the film. 王先生没去。

Besides Mr. Wang，we also went to see the film. 王先生也去了。

Indefinite Tense（一般时态）

一、一般现在时（Present Indefinite Tense）

1．一般现在时通常表示现状、性质、状态和经常性的或习惯性的动作；也可以表示客观事实或普遍真理。如：

（1）I am a teacher. 我是一名教师。

（2）He usually gets up at 7 o'clock. 他通常七点起床。

（3）The sun rises in the east and sets in the west. 太阳东升西落。

（4）Molly enjoys computer games. 莫利喜欢电脑游戏。

（5）There are 60 students in our class. 我们班有 60 名学生。

2．一般现在时通常以动词原形表示；当主语为第三人称单数时，一般在谓语动词原

形后加 -s 或 -es。动词 be 和 have 在第三人称后，变化比较特殊，分别为 am/ is/ are; have/ has。

二、一般过去时（Past Indefinite Tense）

1. 一般过去时表示过去某一时间发生的动作或存在的状态。如：

（1）He was born in 1991. 他 1991 年出生。

（2）The fire broke out during last night. 昨晚火一直烧着。

2. 一般过去时通常由动词过去式表示。不规则动词的过去式有其特殊形式，规则动词的过去式是在动词原形后面加 -d 或 -ed, 具体规则如下：

（1）一般情况下，动词原形加 -ed 构成过去式。如：

play—played，work—worked，want—wanted

（2）如果动词以不发音的 -e 结尾，其过去式的构成为动词原形加 -d。如：

live—lived，hope—hoped，move—moved

（3）如果动词以辅音字母加 -y 结尾，其过去式的构成需要将动词末尾的 -y 变为 -i，再加 -ed。如：

study—studied，cry—cried，try—tried

（4）如果动词是一个以辅音字母结尾的重读闭音节词，其过去式的构成则需双写末尾字母，再加 -ed。如：

stop—stopped，beg—begged，plan—planned

三、一般将来时（Future Indefinite Tense）

一般将来时表示将来发生的动作或状态，主要有以下几种表示法：

1. shall/will+ 动词原形：表示将来发生的动作或状态。如：

（1）I shall leave for Shanghai tomorrow. 明天我将离开上海。

（2）Will you be free this evening? 今晚有空吗？

2. be going to+ 动词原形：常用于口语中，表示主观打算、决心要做的事情或客观上即将要发生的事情。如：

（1）I am going to go shopping this weekend. 本周末我要去逛街。

（2）It's going to rain soon. 很快要下雨。

3. 终止性动词（go，come，leave，start，begin 等）的现在进行时，表示安排或计划好的将要发生的动作。如：

（1）My mother is coming to see me tomorrow. 明天母亲会来看我。

（2）Professor Young is leaving school in one year's time. 杨教授一年后将离开学校。

4. be about to+ 动词原形，表示即将发生的动作。如：

（1）The party is about to begin. 聚会要开始了。

（2）Autumn harvest is about to start. 秋收即将开始。

5. be to+ 动词原形，表示安排或计划好了的动作，含有职责、义务的意味。如：

（1）Mary is to get married next month. 下个月玛丽要结婚了。

（2）We are to meet at the playground. 我们将在操场会面。

Continuous Tense（进行时）

一、现在进行时（Present Continuous Tense）

1. 现在进行时表示此时此刻（说话人说话时）正在进行的动作，它的形式由“be（am/is/ are）+ 现在分词”构成。如：

（1）It is snowing hard outside. 外面雪很大。

（2）I am reading a book. 我正在读书。

2. 现在进行时与 always, constantly 等副词连用时，表示反复出现的或习惯性动作。如：

（1）I'm always losing the way. 我总是迷路。

（2）May is constantly disturbing me. 梅总是不断打搅我。

二、过去进行时（Past Continuous Tense）

1. 过去进行时表示过去某一时刻或某时间段正在进行的动作，它的形式由“was/were+ 现在分词”构成。如：

（1）What were you doing all day yesterday? 你昨天一整天在干什么？

（2）Jane was reading a book when you phoned. 你打电话时珍妮正在看书。

2. 当进行时态用于瞬间动词（leave，come，arrive，stay，go，move 等表示瞬间位置变化的动词），则表达即将发生或预先计划好的活动，翻译成“马上就……”。如：

（1）We are leaving early tomorrow morning. 明天一早我们就动身。

（2）It's beginning to rain. 马上就会下雨。

Present Perfect Tense & Past Perfect Tense（现在完成时和过去完成时）

一、现在完成时

1. 现在完成时表示动作发生在过去，但与现在情况有关系，即用一个发生在过去的动作来说明现在的情况。

2. 现在完成时的构成是“助动词 have/has+ 过去分词”。现在完成时常和 since 所引导的短语或从句或 for 引导的短语连用。由于现在完成时说明的是现在的情况，因此不能和表示过去的时间状语（如 yesterday，last month，three years ago 等）连用。如：

（1）He has gone to Shanghai last week.（×）

（2）We have lived here since 1981.（√）

二、过去完成时

1. 过去完成时表示在过去某一时间或动作以前已经完成了的动作。这个过去的时间可以用 by，before 等介词短语或时间状语从句来表示。

2. 过去完成时的构成是“助动词 had+ 过去分词”。如：

（1）By the end of last week，we had learned ten lessons. 截至上周，我们已经学了 10 课。

（2）Laura had left before I arrived. 我到之前，劳拉已经走了。

三、现在完成时与一般过去时的区别

现在完成时与一般过去时都是表示过去发生的事情，但区别在于：

1. 前者表示动作结果对现在仍有影响，甚至该动作还在继续，而后者表示的动作已经结束，至于是否对现在仍有影响或还在继续，则不得而知。

2. 一般过去时常与表示过去某具体时间的状语连用，现在完成时则不能和明确指出的表示过去某时间的状语（如 yesterday，last week，in 2014，two days ago，just now 等）连用，但可以和不明确指出的表示过去某时间的状语（如 already，yet，sometimes，always，often，recently，once，ever，never）等连用，请比较下面的几组句子：

（1）I have met him. 我已经见过他了。

I met him yesterday. 我昨天看到过他。

（2）He has had lunch. 他吃过午饭了。

He had lunch at 12:00. 他十二点吃的午饭。

（3）I have called to him. 我已经给他打过电话了。

I called to him yesterday. 我昨天给他打过电话。

（4）I have been ill for a week. 我已经生病一周了。（现在还在生病。）

I was ill for a week. 我病了一周。（过去病了一周，现在好了。）

（5）I haven’t seen him for ages. 我好久没有见到他了。

I didn’t see him for ages. 我曾经有好久没见到他（仅指过去。）

单元词汇表

Unit 1

词汇	音标	词性	词义
uniform	/'juːnɪfɔːm/	*n.*	制服
specimen	/'spesɪmɪn/	*n.*	模型人
injection	/ɪn'dʒekʃ(ə)n/	*n.*	注射
etiquette	/'etɪket/	*n.*	礼节
busy	/'bɪzɪ/	*adj.*	忙碌的
major	/'meɪdʒə/	*n.*	主修
certainly	/'səːt(ə)nlɪ/	*adv.*	当然
graduation	/grædʒʊ'eɪʃ(ə)n/	*n.*	毕业
enter	/'entə/	*v.*	进入
knowledge	/'nɒlɪdʒ/	*n.*	知识
drill	/drɪl/	*v.*	训练；钻研
diligently	/'dɪlədʒəntli/	*adv.*	勤奋地
qualification	/ˌkwɒlɪfɪ'keɪʃ(ə)n/	*n.*	资格
register	/'redʒɪstə/	*v.*	登记；注册
lamp	/læmp/	*n.*	灯
instead	/ɪn'sted/	*adv.*	代替；相反
celebrate	/'selɪbreɪt/	*v.*	庆祝；举行
respect	/rɪ'spekt/	*v.*	尊敬
soldier	/'səʊldʒə/	*n.*	军人

词组及专有名词	词义
training classroom	实训室
nursing trolley	护理手推车
practice class	实训课
middle school	中学
head nurse	护士长
junior middle school	高中

at least	至少
in spite of	尽管
grow up	成长
be proud of	自豪
look after	照顾
BP = blood pressure	血压
International Nurses Day	国际护士节
Canada	加拿大
Italy	意大利
Australia	澳大利亚
Germany	德国
England	英格兰
Turkey	土耳其

Unit 2

词汇	音标	词性	词义
visit	/'vɪzɪt/	*v.*	访问；参观；探望
clinic	/'klɪnɪk/	*n.*	诊所；门诊部
pale	/peɪl/	*adj.*	苍白的；无力的
cough	/kɒf/	*v.*	咳嗽
headache	/'hedeɪk/	*n.*	头痛
careful	/'keəfl/	*adj.*	仔细的；小心的
check	/tʃek/	*v.*	检查；核对
serious	/'sɪərɪəs/	*adj.*	严肃的；严重的
advise	/əd'vaɪz/	*v.*	提议；建议
pill	/pɪl/	*n.*	药丸
stomachache	/'stʌməkeɪk/	*n.*	胃痛；腹痛
hamburger	/'hæmbɜːgə/	*n.*	汉堡包
exercise	/'eksəsaɪz/	*v.*	运动；锻炼
hurt	/hɜːt/	*v.*	损害；使受伤
ice	/aɪs/	*n.*	冰

词组及专有名词	词义
keep coughing (keep doing sth.)	一直咳嗽（持续做某事）
all the time	一直；时时刻刻

catch a cold	感冒
as well as	也；又
a large box of …	一大盒……
ice-cream	冰淇淋
fall off	跌落；从……掉下来
lie down	躺下；躺倒
after a while	不久；过一会儿
stay in bed	待在床上；卧床休息

Unit 3

词汇	音标	词性	词义
treatment	/'triːtm(ə)nt/	*n.*	治疗；处理；对待
triage	/'triːaːʒ/	*n.*	分类；分诊
registration	/redʒɪ'streɪʃ(ə)n/	*n.*	登记；注册；挂号
examination	/ɪgˌzæmɪ'neɪʃn/	*n.*	检查
emergency	/ɪ'mɜːdʒ(ə)nsɪ/	*n.*	紧急情况
pharmacy	/'faːməsɪ/	*n.*	药房；药剂学
medical	/'medɪk(ə)l/	*adj.*	内科的；医学的
department	/dɪ'paːtm(ə)nt/	*n.*	部门；系
queuing	/kjuiŋ/	*v.*	排队
lobby	/'lɒbɪ/	*n.*	大堂
embarrassing	/ɪm'bærəsɪŋ/	*adj.*	使人尴尬的
influence	/'ɪnfluəns/	*v.*	影响
local	/'ləʊkl/	*adj.*	当地的
immediately	/ɪ'miːdɪətlɪ/	*adv.*	立即；直接地
elevator	/'elɪveɪtə/	*n.*	电梯
gynecological	/ˌgaɪnɪkə'lɒdʒɪkəl/	*adj.*	妇产科的
affect	/ə'fekt/	*v.*	影响；感染
complain	/kəm'pleɪn/	*v.*	抱怨；发牢骚
mention	/'menʃ(ə)n/	*v.*	谈到；提及
compassion	/kəm'pæʃ(ə)n/	*n.*	同情；怜悯
available	/ə'veɪləb(ə)l/	*adj.*	可得到的
hug	/hʌg/	*v.*	拥抱；紧抱
whisper	/'wɪspə/	*v.*	耳语；低声说出
routine	/ruː'tiːn/	*adj.*	常规的；日常的

supplement	/'sʌplɪm(ə)nt/	*v.*	补充；增补
internship	/'ɪntɜːnʃɪp/	*n.*	实习期

词组及专有名词	词义
queue for	排队
in order to	为了
show up	出现；露面
take one's time	不着急；慢慢来
turn to	转向；变成
prepare sth. for sb.	为某人准备某物
sum up	合计；总结；概括

Unit 4

词汇	音标	词性	词义
syringe	/sɪ'rɪn(d)ʒ/	*n.*	注射器
infusion	/ɪn'fjuːʒ(ə)n/	*n.*	注入
sterilize	/'sterəlaɪz/	*v.*	消毒
insert	/ɪn'sɜːt/	*v.*	插入
needle	/'niːd(ə)l/	*n.*	针
prescription	/prɪ'skrɪpʃ(ə)n/	*n.*	处方
allergic	/ə'lɜːdʒɪk/	*adj.*	过敏的
experience	/ɪk'spɪərɪəns/	*n.*	经验
practice	/'præktɪs/	*n.*	实习
require	/rɪ'kwaɪə/	*v.*	要求
recall	/rɪ'kɔːl/	*v.*	回想
route	/ruːt/	*n.*	途径
competent	/'kɒmpɪtənt/	*adj.*	有能力的
cooperative	/kəʊ'ɒpərətɪv/	*adj.*	合作的
intravenous	/ˌɪntrə'viːnəs/	*adj.*	静脉注射的
drip	/drɪp/	*n.&v.*	点滴；滴下
deliver	/dɪ'lɪvə(r)/	*v.*	传送
fluid	/'fluːɪd/	*n.*	液体
administration	/ədmɪnɪ'streɪʃ(ə)n/	*n.*	管理
overload	/əʊvə'ləʊd/	*v.*	超过负荷
infection	/ɪn'fekʃ(ə)n/	*n.*	感染

词组及专有名词	词义
be allergic to	对……过敏的
refer to...as	把……称为……

Unit 5

词汇	音标	词性	词义
ointment	/'ɒɪntm(ə)nt/	*n.*	药膏；软膏
oxygen	/'ɒksɪdʒ(ə)n/	*n.*	氧；氧气
mask	/mɑːsk/	*n.*	面罩
fair	/feə/	*n.*	集市
cure	/kjʊə(r)/	*n.*	药物；疗法
assistant	/ə'sɪst(ə)nt/	*n.*	助理；助手
forever	/fə'revə/	*adv.*	永远
charge	/tʃɑːdʒ/	*v.*	索价
cancer	/'kænsə/	*n.*	癌症；恶性肿瘤
laboratory	/lə'bɒrətrɪ/	*n.*	实验室
healthy	/'helθɪ/	*adj.*	健康的
release	/rɪ'liːs/	*v.*	释放
poison	/'pɔɪz(ə)n/*n.*	*n.*	毒药
nanometer	/'neɪnəmiːtə/	*n.*	纳米
normal	/'nɔːm(ə)l/	*adj.*	正常的；标准的
surface	/'sɜːfɪs/	*n.*	表面；外表
defense	/dɪ'fens/	*n.*	防卫；抵御
balloon	/bə'luːn/	*n.*	气球
survive	/sə'vaɪv/	*n.*	幸存
test	/test/	*v.*	实验；考察

词组及专有名词	词义
water aqua	水剂
western medicine	西药
drug instruction	药品说明书
herbal medicine	中草药
nano-cell	纳米细胞
as if	似乎；好像
laugh at	嘲笑；蔑视

carry out	执行；进行
fill...with...	装满
cut off	切除；切断
Brufen	布洛芬（药）

Unit 6

词汇	音标	词性	词义
echoscope	/'ekəʊskəʊp/	*n.*	听诊器
lung	/lʌŋ/	*adj.*	肺
arrange	/ə'reɪn(d)ʒ/	*v.*	安排；计划；协商
organ	/'ɔːg(ə)n/	*n.*	器官
annual	/'ænjʊəl/	*adj.*	每年的
ensure	/ɪn'ʃɔː/	*v.*	确保
necessary	/'nesəsərɪ/	*adj.*	必须的；必需品
minor	/'maɪnə(r)/	*adj.*	轻微的
situation	/ˌsɪtjʊ'eɪʃ(ə)n/	*n.*	形势；状况
continuous	/kən'tɪnjʊəs/	*adj.*	连续的
public	/'pʌblɪk/	*adj.*	公众的
clinical	/'klɪnɪkl/	*adj.*	临床的
complete	/kəm'pliːt/	*v.*	完成
refuse	/rɪ'fjuːz/	*v.*	拒绝
refund	/'riːfʌnd/	*v.*	偿还

词组及专有名词	词义
medical examination	体格检查
make an appointment	预约
pulse examination	脉诊
health form	体检表
chest X- ray	胸透
last for	持续
what’s more	而且；更重要的是
be honest to	诚实
have a balance diet	均衡饮食
plan to	计划

more than	多于……
apply for	申请
when it comes to...	谈到……

Unit 7

词汇	音标	词性	词义
check-up	/tʃekʌp/	*v.*	体检；核对；检查
outpatient	/'aʊtpeɪʃ(ə)nt/	*n.*	门诊病人
registration	/ˌredʒɪ'streɪʃ(ə)n/	*n.*	挂号；登记；注册
vomit	/'vɒmɪt/	*v.*	呕吐
urine	/'jʊərɪn/	*n.*	尿；小便
diagnosis	/ˌdaɪəg'nəʊsɪs/	*n.*	诊断
push	/pʊʃ/	*v.*	推；推动
remind	/rɪ'maɪnd/	*v.*	提醒；使想起
medication	/medɪ'keɪʃ(ə)n/	*n.*	药物治疗；药物
itchy	/'ɪtʃɪ/	*adj.*	（使）发痒的
discharge	/dɪs'tʃaːdʒ/	*n.*	出院
symptom	/'sɪm(p)təm/	*n.*	症状；征兆
control	/kən'trəʊl/	*v.*	控制；管理；限制

词组及专有名词	词义
complain of	抱怨；诉苦；诉说症状；主诉
physical examination	身体检查；体检
stay in hospital	待在医院
admission notice	入院通知
payment hall	缴费大厅
advance deposit	预缴押金；定金
call light	呼叫灯
be allergic to...	对……过敏的
short of breath	呼吸短促；呼吸困难；气喘吁吁
look forward to (doing sth.)	期待；期望（做……）
cooperate with	与（某人）协作；合作，配合
Penicillin	青霉素；盘尼西林

Unit 8

词汇	音标	词性	词义
diagnose	/'daɪəgnəʊz/	*v.*	诊断
disinfection	/ˌdɪsɪn'fekʃən/	*n.*	消毒；杀菌
alcohol	/'ælkəhɒl/	*n.*	酒精；酒
uncomfortable	/ʌn'kʌmf(ə)t(ə)b(ə)l/	*adj.*	不舒服、不自在的
hospitalization	/ˌhɒspɪtəlaɪ'zeɪʃən/	*n.*	住院治疗
dizziness	/'dɪzɪnɪs/	*n.*	头晕；眩晕
fecal	/'fiːkəl/	*adj.*	排泄物（渣滓）的
coagulation	/kəʊˌægjʊ'leɪʃən/	*n.*	凝结；凝血
arteriosclerosis	/aːˌtɪərɪəʊsklɪə'rəʊsɪs/	*n.*	动脉硬化
circulation	/sɜːkjʊ'leɪʃ(ə)n/	*n.*	血液循环
relieve	/rɪ'liːv/	*v.*	缓解
optimistic	/ɒptɪ'mɪstɪk/	*adj.*	乐观的
thyroid	/'θaɪrɒɪd/	*n.*	甲状腺
spirit	/'spɪrɪt/	*n.*	精神；心灵
appetite	/'æpɪtaɪt/	*n.*	食欲；嗜好
monitor	/'mɒnɪtə/	*v.*	监视；监督
sodium	/'səʊdɪəm/	*n.*	钠
intake	/'ɪnteɪk/	*n.*	（摄）入量

词组及专有名词	词义
discharging form the hospital	出院
discharge summary	出院小结
doctor in charge	主治医生
ward-round	查房
medication instruction	用药指导
see to	处理；办理
blurred vision	视线模糊
high blood pressure	高血压
be busy with	忙于；从事
before long	不久之后；很快
blood routine	血液常规
chest X-ray	胸部 X 光透视
ECG(Electrocardiograph)	心电图（缩略语）

Neurology	神经内科（学）
Surgery	外科（学）

Unit 9

词汇	音标	词性	词义
traction	/'trækʃ(ə)n/	*n.*	牵引
massage	/mə'sɑːʒ/	*n.*	按摩
recovery	/rɪ'kʌv(ə)rɪ/	*n.*	恢复
choke	/'tʃəʊk/	*v.*	呛；使窒息
absorption	/əb'zɔːpʃ(ə)n/	*n.*	吸收；全神贯注
duty	/'djuːtɪ/	*n.*	责任
overweight	/əʊvə'weɪt/	*adj.*	超重的
stress	/stres/	*v.*	使紧张；强调
obesity	/ə(ʊ)'biːsɪtɪ/	*n.*	肥胖
cause	/kɔːz/	*n.*	原因
grudgingly	/'grʌdʒiŋli/	*adv.*	勉强地
encourage	/ɪn'kʌrɪdʒ/	*v.*	鼓励
abdominal	/æb'dɒmɪn(ə)l/	*adj.*	腹部的
uterus	/'juːt(ə)rəs/	*n.*	子宫
lift	/lɪft/	*v.*	举起
benefit	/'benɪfɪt/	*v.*	有益于
pregnancy	/'pregnənsɪ/	*n.*	怀孕
wound	/wuːnd/	*n.*	伤口
swell	/swel/	*v.*	肿胀；隆起
loose	/luːs/	*adj.*	宽松的

词组及专有名词	词义
supine position	仰卧位
lung capacity	肺活量
balance exercises	平衡练习
blood circulation	血液循环
appendix operation	阑尾手术
intestinal exhaust	肠道排气
pay attention to	注意；重视
too...to...	太……而不能……

lose weight	减肥
high blood pressure	高血压
be harmful to	有害于……
stay up	熬夜
as...as...	像……一样……
try to	试着
cheer up	高兴起来
caesarean section	剖宫产手术
physical and emotional health	身心健康
pelvic floor	骨盆
be kind to	善待
NPO = nothing by mouth	禁食

Unit 10

词汇	音标	词性	词义
stroke	/strəʊk/	*n.*	中风
verbal	/'vɜːb(ə)l/	*adj.*	口头的，言语的
periodical	/pɪərɪ'ɒdɪkl/	*adj.*	周期的，定期的
rehabilitation	/'riːhəˌbɪlɪ'teɪʃən/	*n.*	康复
function	/'fʌŋkʃn/	*n.*	功能，作用
intracerebral	/ˌɪntrəsə'ribrəl/	*adj.*	大脑内的
haemorrhage	/'hemərɪdʒ/	*n.*	出血（尤指大出血）
limb	/lɪm/	*n.*	枝干；肢，翼；大树枝
dysfunction	/dɪs'fʌŋ(k)ʃ(ə)n/	*n.*	机能障碍，机能失调
cerebral	/'serɪbr(ə)l/	*adj.*	脑的；大脑的
infarction	/ɪn'faːkʃ(ə)n/	*n.*	梗死
barely	/'beəlɪ/	*adv.*	仅仅，勉强；几乎不
injury	/'ɪn(d)(ʒ)(ə)rɪ/	*n.*	伤害，损害
recuperation	/rɪkuːpə'reɪʃ(ə)n/	*n.*	恢复；复原
confine	/kən'faɪn/	*v.*	限制；局限于
ideal	/aɪ'diːəl/	*adj.*	理想的，完美的

regain	/rɪ'geɪn/	*v.*	复得，重回；恢复
valid	/'vælɪd/	*adj.*	有效的

词组及专有名词	**词义**
spinal cord	脊髓
cerebral palsy	大脑性瘫痪

词汇索引表

词汇	音标	词性	词义	单元
		A		
abdominal	/æb'dɒmɪn(ə)l/	*adj.*	腹部的	9
absorption	/əb'zɔːpʃ(ə)n/	*n.*	吸收；全神贯注	9
administration	/əd͵mɪnɪ'streɪʃn/	*n.*	管理	4
advise	/əd'vaɪz/	*v.*	提议；建议	2
affect	/ə'fekt/	*v.*	影响；感染	3
alcohol	/'ælkəhɒl/	*n.*	酒精；酒	8
allergic	/ə'lɜːdʒɪk/	*adj.*	过敏的	4
annual	/'ænjuəl/	*adj.*	每年的	6
appetite	/'æpɪtaɪt/	*n.*	食欲；嗜好	8
arrange	/ə'reɪndʒ/	*v.*	安排；计划；协商	6
arteriosclerosis	/ɑː͵tɪərɪəʊsklə'rəʊsɪs/	*n.*	动脉硬化	8
assistant	/ə'sɪstənt/	*n.*	助理；助手	5
available	/ə'veɪləb(ə)l/	*adj.*	可得到的	3
		B		
balloon	/bə'luːn/	*n.*	气球	5
barely	/'beəlɪ/	*adv.*	仅仅，勉强；几乎不	10
benefit	/'benɪfɪt/	*v.*	有益于	9
busy	/'bɪzɪ/	*adj.*	忙碌的	1
		C		
cancer	/'kænsə(r)/	*n.*	癌症；恶性肿瘤	5
careful	/'keəfl/	*adj.*	仔细的；小心的	2
cause	/kɔːz/	*n.*	原因	9
celebrate	/'selɪbreɪt/	*v.*	庆祝；举行	1
cerebral	/'serəbrəl/	*adj.*	脑的；大脑的	10
certainly	/'sɜːt(ə)nlɪ/	*adv.*	当然	1
charge	/tʃɑːdʒ/	*v.*	索价	5

check	/tʃek/	*v.*	检查；核对	2
check-up	/tʃekʌp/	*v.*	体检；核对；检查	7
choke	/'tʃəʊk/	*v.*	呛；使窒息	9
circulation	/ˌsɜːkjə'leɪʃn/	*n.*	血液循环	8
clinic	/'klɪnɪk/	*n.*	诊所；门诊部	2
clinical	/'klɪnɪkl/	*adj.*	临床的	6
coagulation	/kəʊˌægjʊ'leɪʃn/	*n.*	凝结；凝血	8
compassion	/kəm'pæʃ(ə)n/	*n.*	同情；怜悯	3
competent	/'kɒmpɪtənt/	*adj.*	有能力的	4
complain	/kəm'pleɪn/	*v.*	抱怨；发牢骚	3
complete	/kəm'pliːt/	*v.*	完成	6
confine	/kən'faɪn/	*v.*	限制；局限于	10
continuous	/kən'tɪnjuəs/	*adj.*	连续的	6
control	/kən'trəʊl/	*v.*	控制；管理；限制	7
cooperative	/kəʊ'ɒpərətɪv/	*adj.*	合作的	4
cough	/kɒf/	*v.*	咳嗽	2
cure	/kjʊə(r)/	*n.*	药物；疗法	5
		D		
defense	/dɪ'fens/	*n.*	防卫；抵御	5
deliver	/dɪ'lɪvə(r)/	*v.*	传送	4
department	/dɪ'pɑːtm(ə)nt/	*n.*	部门；系	3
diagnose	/'daɪəgnəʊz/	*v.*	诊断	8
diagnosis	/ˌdaɪəg'nəʊsɪs/	*n.*	诊断	7
diligently	/'dɪlədʒəntlɪ/	*adv.*	勤奋地	1
discharge	/dɪs'tʃɑːdʒ/	*n.*	出院	7
disinfection	/ˌdɪsɪn'fekʃən/	*n.*	消毒；杀菌	8
dizziness	/'dɪzɪnəs/	*n.*	头晕；眩晕	8
drill	/drɪl/	*v.*	训练；钻研	1
drip	/drɪp/	*n.&v.*	点滴；滴下	4
duty	/'djuːtɪ/	*n.*	责任	9
dysfunction	/dɪs'fʌŋkʃn/	*n.*	机能障碍，机能失调	10
		E		
echoscope	/'ekəʊskəʊp/	*n.*	听诊器	6

elevator	/'elɪveɪtə(r)/	*n.*	电梯	3
embarrassing	/ɪm'bærəsɪŋ/	*adj.*	使人尴尬的	3
emergency	/ɪ'mɜːdʒ(ə)nsɪ/	*n.*	紧急情况	3
encourage	/ɪn'kʌrɪdʒ/	*v.*	鼓励	9
ensure	/ɪn'ʃʊə(r)/	*v.*	确保	6
enter	/'entə/	*v.*	进入	1
etiquette	/'etɪket/	*n.*	礼节	1
examination	/ɪgˌzæmɪ'neɪʃn/	*n.*	检查	3
exercise	/'eksəsaɪz/	*v.*	运动；锻炼	2
experience	/ɪk'spɪərɪəns/	*n.*	经验	4

F

fair	/feə(r)/	*n.*	集市	5
fecal	/'fiːkl/	*adj.*	排泄物（渣滓）的	8
fluid	/'fluːɪd/	*n.*	液体	4
forever	/fər'evə(r)/	*adv.*	永远	5
function	/'fʌŋkʃn/	*n.*	功能，作用	10

G

graduation	/grædʒʊ'eɪʃ(ə)n/	*n.*	毕业	1
grudgingly	/'grʌdʒɪŋlɪ/	*adv.*	勉强地	9
gynecological	/gaɪnəkə'lɒdʒɪkəl/	*adj.*	妇产科的	3

H

haemorrhage	/'hemərɪdʒ/	*n.*	出血（尤指大出血）	10
hamburger	/'hæmbɜːgə(r)/	*n.*	汉堡包	2
headache	/'hedeɪk/	*n.*	头痛	2
healthy	/'helθɪ/	*adj.*	健康的	5
hospitalization	/ˌhɒspɪtəlaɪ'zeɪʃn/	*n.*	住院治疗	8
hug	/hʌg/	*v.*	拥抱；紧抱	3
hurt	/hɜːt/	*v.*	损害；使受伤	2

I

ice	/aɪs/	*n.*	冰	2
ideal	/aɪ'diːəl/	*adj.*	理想的，完美的	10
immediately	/ɪ'miːdɪətlɪ/	*adv.*	立即；直接地	3
infarction	/ɪn'faːkʃn/	*n.*	梗死形成	10

infection	/ɪn'fekʃn/	*n.*	感染	4
influence	/'ɪnfluəns/	*v.*	影响	3
infusion	/ɪn'fjuːʒn/	*n.*	注入	4
injection	/ɪn'dʒekʃ(ə)n/	*n.*	注射	1
injury	/'ɪndʒərɪ/	*n.*	伤害，损害	10
insert	/ɪn'sɜːt/	*v.*	插入	4
instead	/ɪn'sted/	*adv.*	代替；相反	1
intake	/'ɪnteɪk/	*n.*	（摄）入量	8
internship	/'ɪntɜːnʃɪp/	*n.*	实习期	3
intracerebral	/ɪntrə'serəbrəl/	*adj.*	大脑内的	10
intravenous	/ˌɪntrə'viːnəs/	*adj.*	静脉注射的	4
itchy	/'ɪtʃɪ/	*adj.*	（使）发痒的	7
		K		
knowledge	/'nɒlɪdʒ/	*n.*	知识	1
		L		
laboratory	/lə'bɒrətrɪ/	*n.*	实验室	5
lamp	/læmp/	*n.*	灯	1
lift	/lɪft/	*v.*	举起	9
limb	/lɪm/	*n.*	枝干；肢，翼；大树枝	10
lobby	/'lɒbɪ/	*n.*	大堂	3
local	/'ləʊkl/	*adj.*	当地的	3
loose	/luːs/	*adj.*	宽松的	9
lung	/lʌŋ/	*n.*	肺	6
		M		
major	/'meɪdʒə/	*n.*	主修	1
mask	/maːsk/	*n.*	面罩	5
massage	/mə'saːʒ/	*n.*	按摩	9
medical	/'medɪk(ə)l/	*adj.*	内科的；医学的	3
medication	/ˌmedɪ'keɪʃn/	*n.*	药物治疗；药物	7
mention	/'menʃ(ə)n/	*v.*	谈到；提及	3
minor	/'maɪnə(r)/	*adj.*	轻微的	6
monitor	/'mɒnɪtə(r)/	*v.*	监视；监督	8

refuse	/rɪ'fjuːz/	*v.*	拒绝	6
regain	/rɪ'geɪn/	*v.*	复得，重回；恢复	10
register	/'redʒɪstə/	*v.*	登记；注册	1
registration	/ˌredʒɪ'streɪʃn/	*n.*	挂号；登记；注册	7
registration	/redʒɪ'streɪʃ(ə)n/	*n.*	登记；注册；挂号	3
rehabilitation	/ˌriːəˌbɪlɪ'teɪʃn/	*n.*	康复	10
release	/rɪ'liːs/	*v.*	释放	5
relieve	/rɪ'liːv/	*v.*	缓解	8
remind	/rɪ'maɪnd/	*v.*	提醒；使想起	7
require	/rɪ'kwaɪə(r)/	*v.*	要求	4
respect	/rɪ'spekt/	*v.*	尊敬	1
route	/ruːt/	*n.*	途径	4
routine	/ruː'tiːn/	*adj.*	常规的；日常的	3
		S		
serious	/'sɪərɪəs/	*adj.*	严肃的；严重的	2
situation	/ˌsɪtʃu'eɪʃn/	*n.*	形势；状况	6
sodium	/'səʊdɪəm/	*n.*	钠	8
soldier	/'səʊldʒə/	*n.*	军人	1
specimen	/'spesɪmɪn/	*n.*	模型人	1
spirit	/'spɪrɪt/	*n.*	精神；心灵	8
sterilize	/'sterəlaɪz/	*v.*	消毒	4
stomachache	/'stʌməkeɪk/	*n.*	胃痛；腹痛	2
stress	/stres/	*v.*	使紧张；强调	9
stroke	/strəʊk/	*n.*	中风	10
supplement	/'sʌplɪmənt/	*v.*	补充；增补	3
surface	/'sɜːfɪs/	*n.*	表面；外表	5
survive	/sə'vaɪv/	*v.*	幸存	5
swell	/swel/	*v.*	肿胀；隆起	9
symptom	/'sɪmptəm/	*n.*	症状；征兆	7
syringe	/sɪ'rɪndʒ/	*n.*	注射器	4
		T		
test	/test/	*v.*	实验；考察	5
thyroid	/'θaɪrɔɪd/	*n.*	甲状腺	8

traction	/'trækʃ(ə)n/	*n.*	牵引	9
treatment	/'triːtm(ə)nt/	*n.*	治疗；处理；对待	3
triage	/'triːɑːʒ/	*n.*	分类；分诊	3
		U		
uncomfortable	/ʌn'kʌmftəbl/	*adj.*	不舒服、不自在的	8
uniform	/'juːnɪfɔːm/	*n.*	制服	1
urine	/'jʊərɪn/	*n.*	尿；小便	7
uterus	/'juːt(ə)rəs/	*n.*	子宫	9
		V		
valid	/'vælɪd/	*adj.*	有效的	10
verbal	/'vɜːbl/	*adj.*	口头的，言语的	10
visit	/'vɪzɪt/	*v.*	访问；参观；探望	2
vomit	/'vɒmɪt/	*v.*	呕吐	7
		W		
whisper	/'wɪspə/	*v.*	耳语；低声说出	3
wound	/wuːnd/	*n.*	伤口	9

教学基本要求

一、课程性质和课程任务

英语是世界通用语言之一，是国际交流的重要工具。英语课程是中等职业学校学生必修的一门公共基础课。本课程的任务是：使医护生掌握一定的英语基础知识和基本技能，培养医护生在日常生活和医护场景中的英语语言应用能力；培养医护生的文化意识，提高医护生的思想品德修养和文化素养；为医护生的职业生涯、继续学习和终身发展奠定基础。

二、课程教学目标

中职《医护英语》应从培养初级应用型医护人才的目标出发，结合学生毕业后的工作实际，以“护理技术教学基本要求”为主线，以提示相关医学知识为辅，选择重点护理技术的各个环节和流程，从专业英语词汇、读写能力、听说能力等方面对学生进行训练，为学生提供未来医护工作岗位所需要的医护专业方面的英语基本知识和基本技能。

（一）听

1. 能根据日常生活和职业场景中的多步骤指令做出相应反应；
2. 能理解所听日常交际对话的大意；
3. 能借助图片、图像等听懂职业场景中的简单活动安排和会话。

（二）说

1. 能对日常询问和要求做出恰当反应；
2. 能就日常生活及相关职业话题进行简单交谈；
3. 能运用所学口语进行交际。

（三）读

1. 能根据上下文和构词法猜测词义；
2. 能根据文章信息进行简单的推理、判断；
3. 能根据需要从网络或其他渠道查找信息。

（四）写

1. 能根据提示或关键词转述课文大意；
2. 能简要描述熟悉的事件和经历；
3. 能用英语初步处理简单的常规业务，如接诊、处理业务电话、信函、电子邮件；
4. 能根据范例仿写应用文，如通知、电子邮件、个人履历等。

（五）语音

1. 能根据语音、语调理解日常生活中说话者的意图；
2. 能在交流中做到语音、语调达意。

（六）词汇

学习 1 900 个左右单词（含九年义务教育阶段的词汇），同时学习 200 个左右习惯用语和固定搭配。学习 200 个左右行业通用的专业词汇及缩略语，能根据构词法自主扩展词汇量。

（七）语法

能理解课本附录中语法项目的形式和意义，并能够使用。

三、教学内容和要求

教学内容	教学要求			教学活动参考
	了解	理解	掌握	
Unit 1 Topic: Welcome to the Nursing School				布置并完成任务 理论讲授 多媒体演示 角色扮演 小组讨论 多元评价
Warm-up		✓		
Dialogue			✓	
Reading			✓	
Extensive Reading	✓			
Writing: Personal Data Forms		✓		
Unit 2 Topic: Go to Hospital				布置并完成任务 理论讲授 多媒体演示 角色扮演 小组讨论 多元评价
Warm-up		✓		
Dialogue			✓	
Reading			✓	
Extensive Reading	✓			
Writing: Notices		✓		
Unit 3 Topic: Treatment (Triage)				布置并完成任务 理论讲授 多媒体演示 角色扮演 小组讨论 多元评价
Warm-up		✓		
Dialogue			✓	
Reading			✓	
Extensive Reading	✓			
Writing: Plans		✓		
Unit 4 Topic: Giving Injection				布置并完成任务 理论讲授 多媒体演示 角色扮演 小组讨论 多元评价
Warm-up		✓		
Dialogue			✓	
Reading			✓	
Extensive Reading	✓			
Writing: Personal Letters	✓			

续表

教学内容	教学要求			教学活动参考
	了解	理解	掌握	
Unit 5 Topic: Drug Treatment				布置并完成任务 理论讲授 多媒体演示 角色扮演 小组讨论 多元评价
Warm-up		√		
Dialogue			√	
Reading			√	
Extensive Reading	√			
Writing: E-mails		√		
Unit 6 Topic: Medical Examination				布置并完成任务 理论讲授 多媒体演示 角色扮演 小组讨论 多元评价
Warm-up		√		
Dialogue			√	
Reading			√	
Extensive Reading	√			
Writing: Memos		√		
Unit 7 Topic: Admitted to Hospital				布置并完成任务 理论讲授 多媒体演示 角色扮演 小组讨论 多元评价
Warm-up		√		
Dialogue			√	
Reading			√	
Extensive Reading	√			
Writing: Diary Entries		√		
Unit 8 Topic: Discharging from the Hospital				布置并完成任务 理论讲授 多媒体演示 角色扮演 小组讨论 多元评价
Warm-up		√		
Dialogue			√	
Reading			√	
Extensive Reading	√			
Writing: Nursing Notes		√		
Unit 9 Topic: Health Education				布置并完成任务 理论讲授 多媒体演示 角色扮演 小组讨论 多元评价
Warm-up		√		
Dialogue			√	
Reading			√	
Extensive Reading	√			
Writing: Cover Letters		√		

续表

教学内容	教学要求			教学活动参考
	了解	理解	掌握	
Unit 10 Topic: Rehabilitation Instruction				布置并完成任务 理论讲授 多媒体演示 角色扮演 小组讨论 多元评价
Warm-up		√		
Dialogue			√	
Reading			√	
Extensive Reading	√			
Writing: Resumes		√		

四、学时分配建议（72 学时）

教学内容	学时数				
	Warm-up and Dialogue	Reading	Extensive Reading	Writing	小计
Unit 1	2	2	1	1	6
Unit 2	2	2	1	1	6
Unit 3	2	2	1	1	6
Unit 4	2	2	1	1	6
Unit 5	2	2	1	1	6
Unit 6	2	2	1	1	6
Unit 7	2	2	1	1	6
Unit 8	2	2	1	1	6
Unit 9	2	2	1	1	6
Unit 10	2	2	1	1	6
课堂讲练合计	20	20	10	10	60
复习、考试					8
机动					4

五、教学基本要求说明

（一）适用对象与参考学时

本教学基本要求可供中职护理、助产、药剂、医学检验技术等专业使用，总学时为72，其中课堂讲练 60 学时，复习考试 8 学时，机动 4 学时，教师可根据实际情况制订本校授课计划。

（二）教学要求

本教材每单元由 Section A、Section B、Section C 三个部分组成，包括导入、对话、精读、泛读、写作五大内容。

一、导入部分（Warm-up）：该部分循序渐进地设计了单词搭配、词组辨音、单句理解、对答问答等题型，主要体现主题场景下常见的事物。旨在在训练和提高学生的英语听力基础上，导入单元学习。

二、对话部分（Dialogue）：话题设计紧扣单元主题，通过简单对话落实单元语言目标。着重培养学生用英语进行医护、护患之间对话的能力，突出了本教材的实用性和功能性。对话涵盖单元医护环节的最基本交际用语和内容，并适当增添了一些常用语。

三、精读部分（Reading）：每单元有一篇与主题相关联的精读课文，长度在200～300词之间。课文以本单元交际话题为中心展开，一般为本单元对话内容的补充或延伸。为培养学生正确的阅读方式和习惯，课文以阅读任务导入，并针对课文中的字、词、句型及语法要点，在课文后的阅读理解任务中以不同类型的练习形式全面展示，供教师精讲、学生精读。作为总结，精读部分后设计的语法点对Section A部分的功能用语进行汇总。

四、泛读部分（Extensive Reading）：泛读部分为扩充阅读材料。作为精读文章的拓展部分，泛读部分主要推介相关的医学科普知识，篇幅略长于课文。教学要求以理解为主，旨在帮助学生提高泛读能力。为了帮助学生理解课文，课文以阅读任务导入，并将课文的中心句展示在课文后的阅读任务中。重要的句子结构和语法知识点等在课文注释中进行了详尽的解析。

五、写作部分（Writing）：结合医护生日常生活、学习、工作场景，进行写作训练。主要通过范文，要求学生能够阅读并仿写个人信息表、通知、计划、私人信函、电子邮件、备忘录、护理记录、求职信、求职简历等应用文，并结合医护工作进行仿写练习。

（三）教学建议

1. 在教学过程中积极采用现代化教学手段，加强直观教学，充分发挥教师的主导作用和学生的主体作用。要以学生为本，发挥学生的自主性，建立融洽的师生互动关系，培养学生积极的情感和态度，激发学习兴趣，鼓励学生积极尝试，勇于实践，体验成功，树立自信心。

2. 课堂教学要注重培养学生语言综合应用能力。依据教学内容与要求，结合行业的实际需求，利用真实场景或设置虚拟场景，选择真实或实用的语言材料，设计符合学生实际、目的明确、操作性强、丰富多样的课内外教学活动。引导学生在完成任务的过程中，体验语言，培养技能，积极实践，提高语言综合应用能力。

3. 教师要面向全体学生，因材施教。要尊重学生的差异，为其提供多种学习选择。对基础较薄弱的学生要进行补偿教学，对学有余力的学生要进行拓展教学，适应学生的个性发展需求，使每个学生均学有所得。

4. 教学评价可采用作业、课内外活动、听力测试、口试和笔试等形式，也可采用真实性任务。注重考查学生实际运用语言的能力，兼顾策略、情感和学习态度等对学生进行学习能力、实践能力和应用新知识能力的综合考核，以期达到教学目标提出的各项任务，促进学生发展。

参考答案

Unit 1

Section A

Warm up

Ⅰ. C D F E A B

Ⅱ. 3 2 1 4

Ⅲ.

Mary—is giving an injection.

Nancy—is taking BP.

Nursing Class 1—is practicing nursing etiquette.

We—are having nursing practice class.

Reading

Ⅲ. 1-5 CDBDA 6-10 DCDBD 11 D

Section B

Extensive reading

Ⅲ. 1-5 FFTFT

Section C

First name	Ming	Family name	Zhang	Gender	Male
Nationality	Chinese	Date of Birth	Nov.18th,1998		
Family Address	Room 605, Unit 2, Building No.10, Dehua Road No. 588, Shijicheng Community, Lianxi District. Jiujiang, Jiangxi, P.R.China				
Telephone	0792-255666	Mobile Phone		13312345678	
E-mail	zhangming@163.com	ID/Passport Number		360001199811170011	

Unit 2

Section A

Warm up

Ⅰ. C D F A B E

Ⅱ. 3 1 4 2

Ⅲ.

toothache—see a dentist

fever—take your temperature

cut myself—put some medicine and dress the wound

have a sore throat—drink some hot tea with honey

Reading

Ⅲ. 1-5 BADCB 6-10 ACBCD 11 A

Section B

Extensive reading

Ⅲ. 1-5 FTFTF

Section C

Exercise A

1. Oct. 20th, 2017
2. first aid and emergency treatment
3. Conference Room 301
4. 3 pm,October 20th Friday
5. College of Nursing

Exercise B

1. How to Improve Your Spoken English
2. Amy Powell, Professor of English Department
3. 10 am, September 18th
4. Auditorium
5. Students' Union

Unit 3

Section A

Warm up

Ⅰ. F C E A B D

Ⅱ. 2 1 4 3

Ⅲ.

Mr. Li is queuing for registration—at the lobby on the first floor.

Ms. Chen is getting the medicine—at the pharmacy at the corner.

My sister is waiting to see the doctor—outside the Medical Department.

Doctor Zhang is examining the patient—in the examination room on the second floor.

Reading

Ⅲ. 1-5 CBDAB 6-10 ACDAB

Section B

Extensive reading

Ⅲ. 1-5 TFFTT

Section C

17th-23rd Jul. 2017	Pre-job training
24th Jul.- 23rd Aug. 2017	Emergency Department
24th Aug.- 23rd Sept. 2017	Medical Department
24th Sept.- 23rd Oct. 2017	Surgical Department
24th Oct.- 23rd Nov. 2017	Gynecological Department
24th Nov.- 23rd Dec. 2017	Paediatric Department
24th Dec. 2017-23rd Jan. 2018	Orthopedic Department
24th Jan.- 23rd Feb. 2018	Traditional Chinese Medicine Department
24th Feb.-16th Mar. 2018	Operating Room

Unit 4

Section A

Warm up

Ⅰ. F A B E C D

Ⅱ. 2 4 3 1

Ⅲ.

Emily is careful to—do a skin test.

The boy is scared of—being given an injection.

The child is curious about—being sterilized his skin.

The baby is calm—when the nurse gives him IV fluids.

Reading

Ⅲ. 1-5 BDDCD 6-10 BCACA 11-15 BCDCA

Section B

Extensive reading

Ⅲ. 1-5 FTFFT

Section C

1. looking after/taking care of
2. operation
3. treatment
4. recover
5. responsible

Unit 5

Section A

Warm up

Ⅰ. B A E C F D

Ⅱ. 4 1 3 2

Ⅲ.

Lily should rub the ointment—when she needs.

Julia should read the instruction—before taking the medicine.

Mary should take in oxygen—once a day at bedtime.

Dina should take western medicine—two tablets three times a day on an empty stomach.

Reading

Ⅲ. 1-5 CCBBA 6-10 DCCBA

Section B

Extensive reading

Ⅲ. 1-5 FFFTF

Section C

1. Making an appointment
2. superb skills
3. operation
4. change the dressing
5. on duty

Unit 6

Section A

Warm up

Ⅰ. C F B D A E

Ⅱ. 1 4 2 3

Ⅲ.

Health form filling—begins at 7:00 am.

Chest X-ray—begins at 9:00 am.

Lung's capacity measurement—begins at 8:30 am.

Talking about medical history to doctors—begins at 11:00 am.

Reading

Ⅲ. 1-5 CAADA 6-10 BDABD 11 A

Section B

Extensive reading

Ⅲ. 1-5 TTFTF

Section C

1. In order to
2. how to deal with
3. at 9:00 am
4. No.4 meeting room
5. on time

Unit 7

Section A

Warm up

Ⅰ. E D A B F C

Ⅱ. 3 4 2 1

Ⅲ.

Lily—is writing the nursing notes.

John—is transferring the patient to the Internal Medicine Department.

Linda—is checking the medical records.

Mary—is reserving the hospital beds.

Reading

Ⅲ. 1-5 DCBCA 6-10 BBABC 11 A

Section B

Extensive reading

Ⅲ. 1-5 TFFTF

Section C

Date: October 16th, 2017. Monday Weather: Rainy

1. Michael Smith	2. admitted to	3. vomiting	4. October 16, 2017
5. in hospital	6. improved	7. nausea	
8. according to the doctor's advice		9. medications	10. after discharge

Unit 8

Section A

Warm up

Ⅰ. D E F A B C

Ⅱ. 1 3 2 4

Ⅲ.

makes a ward-round— from 9:00 am to 10:00 am

gives medication instructions— before the patients leave the hospital

completes discharge summaries—after the ward-round

tidy up the wards—after the patients leave the hospital

Reading

Ⅲ. 1-5 DCDBC 6-10 DCCBA

Section B

Extensive reading

Ⅲ. 1-5 FFFFT

Section C

<table>
<tr><th colspan="7">Nursing Notes</th></tr>
<tr><td colspan="2">Name</td><td>Li Yue</td><td>Age</td><td>45</td><td>Gender</td><td>Male</td></tr>
<tr><td colspan="2">Department</td><td>Surgery</td><td>Bed No.</td><td>13</td><td>Admission Number</td><td>1703051</td></tr>
<tr><td colspan="3">Date & Time</td><td colspan="2">10:00 July 18th, 2017</td><td colspan="2"></td></tr>
<tr><td rowspan="4">Vital signs</td><td>Temperature</td><td>℃</td><td colspan="2">36.2</td><td colspan="2"></td></tr>
<tr><td>Pulse</td><td>Time/min</td><td colspan="2">76</td><td colspan="2"></td></tr>
<tr><td>Respiratory</td><td>Time/min</td><td colspan="2">18</td><td colspan="2"></td></tr>
<tr><td>Blood Pressure</td><td>mmHg</td><td colspan="2">120/80</td><td colspan="2"></td></tr>
<tr><td colspan="2">SpO2</td><td>%</td><td colspan="2">99</td><td colspan="2"></td></tr>
<tr><td colspan="3">Catheter and drainage tube</td><td colspan="2">✓</td><td colspan="2"></td></tr>
<tr><td>Intake</td><td colspan="2">Volume ml</td><td colspan="2">800</td><td colspan="2"></td></tr>
<tr><td>Output</td><td colspan="2">Volume ml</td><td colspan="2">200</td><td colspan="2"></td></tr>
<tr><td colspan="3">Others</td><td colspan="2"></td><td colspan="2"></td></tr>
<tr><td colspan="3">Signature</td><td colspan="2"></td><td colspan="2"></td></tr>
<tr><td colspan="7">Explanation: If nothing has been observed, sign the blank with "N" .</td></tr>
</table>

Unit 9

Section A

Warm up

Ⅰ. C D B A E F

Ⅱ. 3 1 2 4

Ⅲ.

sleep in supine position—to avoid choke

eat fluids—to be easy for absorption

be in traction—to help the recovery

go for a massage—to promote the blood circulation

Reading

Ⅲ. 1-5 DAABD 6-10 CDADC

Section B

Extensive Reading

Ⅲ. 1-5 FTFTT

Section C

1. Dear Mr. Wang
2. job ad/ want ad(advertisement)
3. I will graduate from nursing school
4. I has been a student nurse in the First Hospital

5. the copy of my Graduation Certificate

6. Please let me hear from you as soon as possible

Unit 10

Section A

Warm up

Ⅰ. F C E A B D

Ⅱ. 4 3 2 1

Ⅲ.

Bob's grandfather—is giving acupuncture a whirl.

Mr. Mark—is helping his wife with physical training.

Mary's mother—is cooling Mary's head with a cold towel.

Mr. Black—is practicing walking with a walker.

Reading

Ⅲ. 1-5 BCACD 6-10 DDACA

Section B

Extensive Reading

Ⅲ. 1-5 FTFTT

Section C

略